2 FAT

2

FLY

350 lbs Down

- No Surgery, No Pills, No Injections -

By

Quanjay Jones

Copyrights

This book is published by:
Colby Bear Media LLC,
Columbia, SC, USA
ISBN: 978-1-7331159-6-4

Colby Bear Media LLC
Email: **ColbyBearMediaSC@gmail.com**

Legal & Medical Disclaimer

This book is for **informational and educational purposes only** and is not intended as a substitute for medical, nutritional, psychological, or professional advice. The author and publisher make no representations or warranties regarding the accuracy, applicability, or completeness of the contents of this book. **Readers are encouraged to consult a licensed medical or mental health professional before making any changes to their health, diet, or exercise routines.** Any reliance on the information provided is solely at the reader's discretion and risk. The author and publisher disclaim any liability for any injuries, losses, or damages incurred as a result of the application of any advice or strategies contained in this book.

Design & Production Credits
Editor: Quanjay Jones
Cover Design: Quanjay Jones
Formatting & Layout: Quanjay Jones
Printed & Distributed by
Colby Bear Media LLC
Printed in the United States of America

Environmental Responsibility

This book has been printed using environmentally responsible practices. The publisher supports sustainable printing efforts and encourages recycling books that are no longer in use.

Author Contact & Social Media
For updates, additional content, and other books by the author, please visit:
colbybearmediasc@gmail.com

2 FAT 2 FLY

Important Disclaimer:

Consult with a Medical Professional Before Starting Any Workout or Diet Plan

Before beginning any workout or diet plan, it is strongly recommended that you consult with a licensed healthcare provider, including your doctor or a qualified medical professional. The information provided in this workbook, including the exercises and nutrition guidelines, is intended for general informational purposes only and is not intended as medical advice.

I am **Quanjay Joculb Jones**, a certified personal trainer, but I am not a medical doctor, a licensed healthcare provider, or a registered dietitian. While I have professional training and experience in fitness and wellness, it's important to understand that any workout program or diet plan can affect individuals differently, and there may be underlying health conditions that need to be addressed prior to engaging in any physical activity or making dietary changes.

Always Seek Professional Guidance:

Physical Health: If you are pregnant, have any existing medical conditions (such as heart disease, diabetes, high blood pressure, joint issues, or previous injuries), or have any concerns about your physical health, it is essential to seek medical advice before starting a new exercise regimen or making significant changes to your diet.

Dietary Concerns: If you have any food allergies, intolerances, or specific dietary needs, consult a licensed nutritionist or dietitian to tailor a plan suited to your unique health requirements.

Mental Health: If you are experiencing mental health challenges that affect your motivation, energy, or ability to focus on a fitness or diet plan, consider seeking support from a mental health professional. Your mental well-being is just as important as your physical health.

Liability:

By engaging with this content, you acknowledge that I, Quanjay Joculb Jones, am not liable for any injuries, health complications, or adverse effects that may arise from following the workout routines or diet recommendations provided in this book. Any exercises or meal plans should be undertaken at your own risk. The information and advice contained in this workbook are not a substitute for professional medical or nutritional guidance.

It is important to listen to your body. If you feel any pain or discomfort during exercise or while making dietary changes, stop immediately and consult a medical professional. It is crucial to adapt the program to your individual abilities, fitness level, and health status. Your health and safety are my top priority, and I strongly encourage you to approach any new fitness or dietary plan with caution and respect for your body's unique needs.

Stay Safe, Stay Healthy, and Always Consult a Professional First!

Dedication

This book is dedicated to every person who has ever suffered because of their weight to those who have felt unseen, unheard, or unworthy because of how the world has judged them. To those who have endured the pain of rejection, the whispers of ridicule, or the silent battle of self-doubt. To those who have struggled with their reflection, felt trapped in their own bodies, or believed that they were anything less than enough.

This is for the ones who have fought against the weight of not just their bodies, but their emotions, their past, and the expectations placed upon them. For those who have turned to food for comfort, to silence the pain, or to fill a void they didn't know how to heal. For those who have felt the sting of discrimination, the burden of health struggles, or the exhaustion of trying, failing, and trying again.

You are more than the number on a scale. You are worthy of love, healing, and a life that feels good inside and out. This book is a testament to your strength, a reminder that change is possible, and a promise that your story does not end in struggle; it begins anew in power, resilience, and self-love. May this book be a light in your journey, guiding you toward healing, renewal, and the realization that you are enough exactly as you are, in this moment, and in every step forward.

Table of Contents

Introduction

I approached the heliport, a mix of excitement and nervousness flooding over me. The helicopter, with its sleek body and spinning rotors, waited on the pad, ready for the journey ahead. The pilot greeted me with a friendly smile as he helped me into my seat and secured my harness. The interior is surprisingly cozy, with large windows offering panoramic views.

The engine roars to life, and the rotors spin faster, creating a rhythmic thumping sound that reverberates through my body. We lift off the ground gently at first, then more steadily, as if the earth itself is letting go of its grip on us. I feel slight pressure as we ascend, and my heart races with the realization that we're actually airborne.

Looking out the window, I see the city below shrinking rapidly. Buildings and streets, once towering and bustling, now look like intricate patterns on a quilt. The sense of perspective is both humbling and exhilarating. As we gain altitude, the pilot points out landmarks below. The familiar shapes of parks and stadiums take on new dimensions from this vantage point. Rivers and highways become winding ribbons, and the sprawling urban landscape gives way to patches of greenery and open spaces.

The helicopter glides smoothly through the sky, and I find myself relaxing into the experience. The horizon stretches out endlessly, a beautiful blend of blue sky and wispy clouds. Sunlight filters through the glass, casting a warm glow inside the cabin. I can see for miles, taking in vistas that stretch far beyond what is visible from the ground.

We fly over rolling hills and forests, the trees below forming a dense, green carpet. Occasionally, the pilot tilts the helicopter, giving me a better view of a particular sight. The sensation of banking and turning is both thrilling and graceful, a dance in the sky.

The sound of the rotors is a constant backdrop, but inside the cabin, it's quieter than I expected. Through the headset, the pilot's voice is clear as he explains what we're seeing and shares stories about the area. His knowledge and passion for flying add another layer of enjoyment to the trip.

As we approach a mountain range, the terrain changes dramatically. Jagged peaks rise majestically, capped with snow even in summer. The helicopter hovers for a moment, allowing me to fully appreciate the stunning landscape. The sheer scale and beauty of the mountains leave me in awe.

As good as that experience sounds, I wish it was my story. Instead, I was forced to sit on a bench as I watched the person I came with climb into the helicopter. The lady at the desk told us that the maximum weight capacity was two hundred and eighty pounds, and I was clearly over that, weighing in at four hundred and eighty-five pounds (485 lbs). I sat on the bench, wanting her not to go, not to leave me there, leave me like everyone else. I started to reminisce and think about my life experiences, all that I had gone through because of being overweight, and in that moment I had a stark realization; then I zoned out, thinking about my childhood.

Growing up in a low-income neighborhood, it was a constant struggle. The house we had through Section 8 was nestled in a rundown part of town and was always bustling with activity. My mom worked multiple jobs to keep us afloat; my stepdad was an alcoholic, and my siblings and I learned to make do with what little we had. Amid all this chaos, I often felt like an outsider, not just because of our financial struggles, but because I was different in another way: I was a fat kid.

School was supposed to be a place of learning and growth, but for me, it was often a place of torment. From the moment I stepped off the bus, the taunts and jeers would start. "Fatso," "Tubby," and "Piggy" were names that varied, but the cruelty behind them was always the same. Classmates would snicker when I walked by, and some even went out of their way to make my life miserable. They'd knock my books out of my hands, trip me in the hallways, and make cruel jokes at my expense. The bullying wasn't just verbal; it was physical and emotional, too.

Lunchtime was especially tough. I'd sit alone at a table, trying to eat my meager lunch as quickly as possible to avoid the stares and whispers. I envied the other kids who seemed to fit in so effortlessly, who laughed and talked without a care in the world. My weight wasn't just a source of ridicule; it was a barrier that kept me isolated, reinforcing the feeling that I didn't belong.

The weight itself was partly due to the lack of nutritious food options available to us. We couldn't afford fresh fruits and vegetables, and fast food was often the most convenient and affordable option. It was a vicious cycle of unhealthy eating habits leading to weight gain, which then led to more bullying, driving me to seek comfort in food even more.

Home was supposed to be my refuge, but even there, the challenges were numerous. My mom, though loving and supportive, was often too exhausted from her multiple jobs, or trying to keep my stepfather off the corner, spending up all the money to give me the attention I craved. My siblings had their own struggles, and while we were close, they couldn't fully understand the depth of my pain that came from things I didn't tell my mom.

As a child, I was forced into a reality I never asked for, a reality that twisted the innocence of my youth into something dark and painful. It was during these early years that my body began to change in ways I couldn't control, and the weight I gained wasn't just physical; it was a weight of trauma, of fear, and of shame that I carried with me every day.

The sexual abuse, the molestation by two guys and two girls, left scars deeper than any physical wound could. My sense of self was shattered, and the weight I gained became my armor, my shield against the world that had hurt me so deeply. Food became my comfort, my escape from the torment that lived in my mind. At first, it felt like a relief a temporary fix to numb the pain. Each bite I took gave me a sense of control, a way to cope with the overwhelming emotions that flooded me.

It didn't matter that the food didn't make the pain go away; it only seemed to provide a moment of peace, a fleeting distraction. I wasn't thinking about the reality of what was happening to me, or the truth about how my body was changing. I just wanted to survive, to keep going, to feel something other than the rage and sadness that consumed me. But as I grew older, the weight didn't just change my body; it changed how people saw me.

It altered my interactions with others and my place in the social structure. I was no longer seen as just another kid; I became the overweight, insecure one, the one who didn't fit in. At school, I was the target of ridicule and judgment, and with every insult, I sank further into myself. The heaviness I felt physically mirrored the emotional burden I carried, and I began to see my body as the enemy, a constant reminder of the trauma I couldn't escape. I began to believe that the only way to cope with the rejection and the shame was to keep feeding the hurt.

With each meal, I could pretend I was fine; I could convince myself that I wasn't broken. But deep down, I knew I wasn't okay. I wasn't just trying to fill the emptiness with food; I was trying to silence the voice in my head that kept reminding me of the horrors I'd endured. I didn't know how to heal, how to confront what had been done to me. So, I fed my pain, watched it grow, and turned a blind eye to the damage. As the years went by, I found that food wasn't just a coping mechanism; it became my identity.

I stopped looking at myself in the mirror because the reflection staring back at me was someone I didn't recognize. I wasn't just overweight; I was carrying the weight of my past. The abuse I had suffered at the hands of those who were supposed to protect me now controlled my every thought, my every action. I became isolated, pulling away from relationships and social situations, convinced that no one would ever accept me for who I was broken, scarred, and carrying too much.

I kept to myself, hiding behind the food, using it as a shield to protect me from the world that had hurt me. But no matter how much I ate, it never seemed to fill the emptiness inside. It was as though I was constantly searching for something to make me feel whole again, but I never found it. I watched my body change, grow larger, and felt more trapped than ever. The weight wasn't just in my stomach; it was in my heart, my soul, and it felt like I would never be free from it. There were moments when I tried to fight against it, when I'd tell myself I would lose the weight, get healthier, and be stronger. But the cycle always pulled me back. I'd start to feel hopeful, only to find myself facing the same pain again, turning to food once more. It was a never-ending struggle, a battle between the desire to heal and the temptation to bury my feelings in food. I had no idea how to break the chains of my past or how to love myself again.

One day, after a particularly harsh incident at school, I came home and broke down in tears. My mom found me in my room, and for the first time, I opened up about everything the bullying, the loneliness, the hopelessness I felt, but I didn't tell her about the molestation because I had been threatened with death if I said anything, and I believed him. I thought that because he said he'd kill me and my family, then the others would do the same. My mom hugged me tightly and told me something I will never forget:

"You are stronger than you know. Don't let them define who you are, son..."

I zoned back in as the tears continued to roll down my eyes. The helicopter began to disappear into the distance, and it was at that moment that I realized that I was too fat to do something as simple as fly on a helicopter ride. And if I didn't do something about it, I was going to miss out on living life due to all of my unhealthy choices. That day, I didn't get to experience what it was like to fly and journey through the sky, but I did experience a journey that would change my life, one that began in my mind and my body.

The journey was far from easy, and there were many setbacks along the way. But with each challenge, I grew stronger and more resilient. The adversity I faced as a poor, fat, black kid taught me valuable lessons about perseverance, self-worth, and the importance of loving myself.

Today, I look back on those difficult years with a sense of pride. **At my heaviest, I was over six hundred pounds (600 lbs)**. I survived and thrived despite the odds stacked against me. I didn't have weight loss surgery, take pills, or shots, though there's nothing wrong with getting help. I chose the natural way, and I'm no longer defined by my past or the cruel words of bullies. Instead, I am defined by my strength, my courage, and my unwavering determination to overcome adversity. My story is one of triumph over hardship, a testament to the power of resilience and the belief that no matter how tough life gets, we have the power to change our destiny.

I talk about my journey because losing weight is a journey that encompasses much more than just the numbers on a scale. It's about transforming your lifestyle, adopting healthier habits, and ultimately improving your overall well-being. This book aims to guide you through the process of weight loss in a sustainable and healthy way, in the hopes that you will finally reach your weight-loss goal.

It's not just about losing weight, but it's about doing it in a healthy and productive way that works best for you; so let's talk about the importance of maintaining a healthy weight. Maintaining a healthy weight is crucial for overall health. It can reduce the risk of chronic diseases such as heart disease, diabetes, and certain cancers. Additionally, achieving a healthy weight can enhance your energy levels, improve your mood, and boost your confidence.

Maintaining a healthy weight has been a personal journey of discovery and resilience for me. It's not just about appearance; it's about nurturing my well-being and embracing life to the fullest. By achieving and maintaining a healthy weight, I've experienced profound improvements in both my physical and mental health. It's given me the energy to pursue my passions and engage fully in the activities that bring me joy.

Physically, maintaining a healthy weight has reduced my risk of chronic diseases such as heart disease, diabetes, and high blood pressure. It's allowed me to move with greater ease and comfort, enhancing my overall mobility and fitness. I've learned that a healthy weight isn't just a number on a scale; it's a foundation for a vibrant, active life.

Emotionally, achieving a healthy weight has boosted my self-esteem and confidence. It's reshaped my body image and liberated me from the insecurities that once weighed me down. Feeling good in my own skin has translated into improved mental well-being, reducing stress and anxiety. It's empowered me to approach life with positivity and resilience, knowing that I'm taking proactive steps to care for myself.

"""Maintaining a healthy weight isn't always easy, but the benefits are profound and far-reaching. It's not just about longevity, though that's important; it's about living each day with vitality and vigor. By prioritizing nutrition, staying active, and making mindful lifestyle choices, I've discovered a path to sustained health and happiness. This journey has taught me that investing in my health is one of the greatest gifts I can give myself, ensuring a future filled with vitality and well-being.

Your Journey Starts Here

The path to weight loss is personal and unique to each individual. It's important to approach this journey with patience, dedication, and an open mind. This book is divided into several parts, each focusing on different aspects of weight loss, from understanding the science behind it to implementing practical nutrition and exercise strategies, and addressing lifestyle changes that support your goals.

By the end of this book, you will have a comprehensive understanding of what it takes to lose weight healthily and sustainably."""" More importantly, you'll be equipped with the tools and knowledge to make lasting changes that enhance your quality of life. Let's begin this journey together.

Chapter 1

Misconceptions Of Weight Loss

Misconceptions About Weight Loss

There are countless myths and misconceptions about weight loss. I had heard many things and believed a lot of them until I did my own research; here's what I found. Many people believe that drastic diets or intense exercise regimens are the only ways to lose weight, but these approaches are often unsustainable and can lead to disappointment and frustration.

Navigating the landscape of weight loss can be daunting, especially with the myriad misconceptions that abound. From crash diets promising quick fixes to the belief that all calories are equal, separating fact from fiction is essential for achieving sustainable results and maintaining overall health.

One common misconception is the effectiveness of crash diets. In my own journey, I've learned firsthand that rapid weight loss through extreme calorie restriction is not only unsustainable but can also be detrimental to health. These diets often lead to muscle loss, nutrient deficiencies, and a slowed metabolism, making it harder to maintain weight loss in the long run.

Another prevalent myth is that all calories are created equal. While calorie intake is important for weight management, the quality of those calories matters just as much. Opting for nutrient-dense foods like fruits, vegetables, and whole grains over processed foods high in sugars and unhealthy fats can significantly impact both weight loss and overall health.

Weight loss supplements are another area ripe with misconceptions. Many claim to enhance metabolism or burn fat, but their safety and efficacy are often questionable. Through my research, I've found that relying on supplements alone is not a sustainable approach to weight loss and can pose risks to health due to potential side effects and interactions with medications.

Carbohydrates often get a bad rap in weight loss discussions, with some believing that they must be avoided entirely. However, carbohydrates are an essential source of energy, and the focus should be on choosing complex carbs that provide sustained energy and essential nutrients. Balancing carbohydrate intake with protein and healthy fats can support weight loss efforts while promoting overall well-being.

Spot reduction is another misconception I've encountered. Despite the desire to target specific areas for fat loss through exercises like crunches or sit-ups, weight loss occurs systematically across the body. Adopting a comprehensive approach that includes cardio, strength training, and a balanced diet is key to achieving overall body fat reduction.

The belief that weight loss is solely a matter of willpower overlooks the complex interplay of factors influencing body weight. Genetics, hormones, metabolism, environment, and lifestyle habits all play significant roles. My journey has taught me that sustainable weight loss requires a holistic approach that addresses these factors through consistent, healthy behaviors such as nutritious eating, regular physical activity, adequate sleep, and effective stress management.

Another common myth is the idea that skipping meals, particularly breakfast, can aid in weight loss. In reality, skipping meals can disrupt metabolism, leading to fluctuations in blood sugar levels and increased cravings later in the day. This can result in overeating and difficulty maintaining a healthy weight over time. Instead, focusing on balanced meals and snacks throughout the day can help regulate hunger, energy levels, and overall calorie intake.

Exercise is often touted as a primary method for weight loss, but the misconception lies in thinking that exercise alone is sufficient. While physical activity is crucial for overall health and can contribute to weight loss by burning calories and building muscle, it is most effective when combined with dietary changes. Without a balanced diet that supports a calorie deficit, achieving significant weight loss solely through exercise can be challenging.

Detox diets and cleanses are another area of misunderstanding in weight loss. These programs often promise to "cleanse" the body of toxins and promote rapid weight loss. However, there is limited scientific evidence to support their effectiveness for long-term weight management or overall health benefits. These diets typically involve severe calorie restriction and may lead to dehydration, nutrient deficiencies, and a slowed metabolism.

A common misconception among individuals seeking weight loss is that it's necessary to eat less and exercise more. While creating a calorie deficit through a combination of reduced calorie intake and increased physical activity is fundamental to weight loss, extreme measures can backfire. Severely restricting calories or over-exercising can lead to fatigue, nutrient deficiencies, and metabolic slowdown, making it harder to sustain weight loss over time.

Lastly, there is a misconception that losing weight means giving up all favorite foods or adopting a restrictive diet. In reality, sustainable weight loss involves finding a balance that includes occasional indulgences and enjoying foods in moderation. Restrictive diets that eliminate entire food groups or label foods as "good" or "bad" can lead to feelings of deprivation and increase the likelihood of binge eating or emotional eating behaviors.

Understanding and addressing these misconceptions can empower individuals to make informed decisions about their weight loss journey. By focusing on sustainable, evidence-based approaches that prioritize overall health and well-being, it is possible to achieve and maintain a healthy weight while enjoying a balanced and fulfilling lifestyle. The next thing I learned was how weight loss works, so let's get into it.

Chapter 2

THE MATH OF NUTRIENTS

Learning the Hard Way: A Wake-Up Call About Nutrient Deficiencies

There was a time in my life when I didn't fully understand the importance of proper nutrition. I knew I had to eat to fuel my body, but I didn't realize that what I put in my body could either nourish me or contribute to my downfall. I learned this lesson the hard way when I was hospitalized due to severe nutrient deficiencies.

It started with feeling unusually fatigued, getting sick more often, and struggling with muscle weakness. At first, I thought it was just part of the daily grind something that would pass. But it didn't. I found myself in a hospital bed, being told by doctors that my body was lacking key nutrients necessary for basic functions.

The deficiencies were severe, affecting everything from my immune system to my energy levels. I had never realized that something as simple as lacking essential vitamins and minerals could cause such a cascade of issues. I learned that without proper nutrients, no amount of willpower or exercise could truly fuel my body or keep me healthy.

That wake-up call was a turning point. I realized that true wellness isn't just about losing weight or hitting fitness goals; it's about understanding how vital it is to nourish your body from the inside out. No more neglecting my body with empty calories or ignoring the nutrients that keep me strong. I began to educate myself on the critical role of vitamins, minerals, and other essential nutrients, and made a commitment to nourish my body properly every day.

This experience not only changed the way I approached my diet and fitness but also helped me realize that a well-balanced, nutrient-dense diet is key to long-term health, not just weight loss. I now understand that good health starts with what we feed our bodies, and that proper nutrition fuels both our physical and mental resilience.

This journey has been one of learning, healing, and empowerment, and I want others to know that it's never too late to start making those changes. The lesson I learned in the hospital wasn't just about eating more; it was about eating right. And that's the message I hope to pass on to you.

Macro-nutrients: Proteins, Carbs, and Fats

Proteins

One of the first things I did when I learned how to properly lose weight was to understand exactly how food is processed in the first place, so we will start with the basics. Proteins are essential macronutrients that play a crucial role in nearly every function of the human body, including muscle growth, tissue repair, enzyme and hormone production, and immune system support. They are made up of amino acids, some of which are essential and must be obtained through diet.

Consuming adequate protein has several positive effects, such as supporting muscle development, enhancing metabolism, helping with weight management, and aiding in cell regeneration and wound healing. Additionally, proteins help regulate important bodily processes, such as oxygen transport and blood sugar balance.

However, excessive protein intake can have negative effects, including kidney strain in individuals with preexisting kidney conditions, an increased risk of dehydration, digestive issues such as bloating and constipation, and potential links to heart disease if consuming too much processed or high-fat animal protein.

The best sources of protein for human consumption are lean meats (chicken, turkey, and fish), eggs, dairy, plant-based proteins (such as lentils, chickpeas, tofu, quinoa, and nuts), and high-quality protein powders made from a plant source. These sources provide essential amino acids while being lower in unhealthy fats and additives.

On the other hand, the worst protein sources include heavily processed meats such as sausages, bacon, and hot dogs, as they are high in saturated fats, sodium, and preservatives, which may increase the risk of chronic diseases such as heart disease and cancer. Ultimately, a well-balanced intake of high-quality proteins from both animal and plant sources supports optimal health and overall well-being.

Carbohydrates

Carbohydrates are the body's primary source of energy, providing fuel for the brain, muscles, and other vital organs. They are broken down into glucose, which is used for immediate energy or stored for later use. Carbohydrates play an essential role in maintaining proper bodily functions, including digestion, metabolism, and overall energy balance.

The positive effects of consuming carbohydrates include sustained energy levels, improved cognitive function, better digestive health (especially from fiber-rich sources), and enhanced athletic performance. They also help regulate blood sugar levels when consumed in their natural, unprocessed forms. However, there are negative effects associated with excessive or poor-quality carbohydrate intake.

Consuming too many refined carbohydrates, such as white bread, sugary drinks, and processed snacks, can lead to weight gain, blood sugar spikes, an increased risk of type 2 diabetes, and heart disease. Overconsumption of simple sugars may also cause energy crashes, cravings, and digestive discomfort. The best sources of carbohydrates for human consumption are whole foods like fruits, vegetables, whole grains (such as brown rice, quinoa, and oats), legumes, and fiber-rich foods. These provide essential nutrients, fiber, and slow-releasing energy, which support overall health.

In contrast, the worst sources of carbohydrates are refined and processed foods like white bread, pastries, candy, sugary cereals, and soda. These offer little nutritional value, contribute to rapid blood sugar fluctuations, and may lead to long-term health problems. Choosing complex, fiber-rich carbohydrates over refined ones ensures better energy levels, improved digestion, and long-term wellness.

Fats

Fats are an essential macro-nutrient that play a vital role in overall health by providing long-term energy, supporting cell growth, protecting organs, and aiding in the absorption of fat-soluble vitamins (A, D, E, and K). They also contribute to brain function, hormone production, and maintaining healthy skin and hair.

The positive effects of consuming healthy fats include improved heart health, better cognitive function, reduced inflammation, and sustained energy levels. Healthy fats, particularly unsaturated fats, help lower bad cholesterol (LDL) while raising good cholesterol (HDL), reducing the risk of cardiovascular disease.

However, excessive fat consumption or eating unhealthy fats can have negative effects on health. Trans fats and excessive saturated fats, found in processed and fried foods, can contribute to high cholesterol, obesity, heart disease, and inflammation. Overconsumption of any fat, even healthy fats, can lead to weight gain due to its high-calorie content.

The best sources of fat include unsaturated fats from avocados, nuts, seeds, olive oil, and fatty fish like salmon and sardines, as well as moderate amounts of healthy saturated fats from sources like coconut oil and grass-fed butter. These fats provide essential nutrients while supporting heart and brain health.

On the other hand, the worst sources of fat are trans fats and highly processed fats found in margarine, fried fast food, processed snacks, and hydrogenated oils. These fats are associated with inflammation, insulin resistance, and an increased risk of chronic diseases. Choosing high-quality, natural fats while avoiding heavily processed fats can help maintain overall well-being and prevent various health issues.

Importance of Micro-nutrients

Micro-nutrients, which include vitamins and minerals, are essential for maintaining overall health and supporting various bodily functions, such as immune response, metabolism, bone health, and brain function. Unlike macronutrients, they are needed in smaller amounts, but their impact on health is significant.

The positive effects of consuming adequate micronutrients include improved immune function, enhanced energy production, stronger bones, better cognitive function, and protection against chronic diseases. For example, vitamin C boosts immunity and supports collagen production, while calcium and vitamin D strengthen bones.

Iron is crucial for oxygen transport in the blood, and B vitamins help convert food into energy. However, micronutrient imbalances can have negative effects on health. Deficiencies in essential vitamins and minerals can lead to serious health issues, such as anemia (iron deficiency), weakened immunity (vitamin C or zinc deficiency), brittle bones (calcium and vitamin D deficiency), and fatigue (B-vitamin deficiency).

On the other hand, excessive intake of certain micronutrients, especially through supplements, can cause toxicity. For example, too much vitamin A can lead to liver damage, and excessive iron intake may result in digestive issues or organ damage. The best sources of micronutrients are whole, nutrient-dense foods like fruits, vegetables, lean proteins, whole grains, nuts, and seeds.

These foods provide a variety of vitamins and minerals in their most bioavailable forms. The worst sources are processed foods and fast foods, which often lack essential nutrients and may contain artificial additives, unhealthy fats, and excessive sodium, leading to nutrient deficiencies over time. A balanced diet rich in natural, whole foods ensures proper micronutrient intake, supporting long-term health and overall well-being.

Common Deficiencies

Common deficiencies can have significant effects on overall health, as they deprive the body of essential nutrients needed for proper functioning. Deficiencies in key vitamins and minerals can lead to a variety of health issues, impacting energy levels, immune function, cognitive health, and overall well-being. The positive effects of addressing these deficiencies include improved energy, stronger immunity, better mental clarity, enhanced muscle and bone strength, and overall disease prevention.

Ensuring adequate intake of essential nutrients supports long-term health and prevents complications related to malnutrition. However, when deficiencies are left untreated, they can have negative effects on the body. For example, iron deficiency can cause anemia, leading to fatigue, weakness, and pale skin. Vitamin D deficiency may result in weakened bones, joint pain, and an increased risk of osteoporosis.

A lack of B vitamins can cause neurological issues, mood disorders, and low energy, while insufficient vitamin C can lead to a weakened immune system and slow wound healing. The best sources of essential nutrients come from a well-balanced diet that includes a variety of whole foods. Iron-rich foods such as lean meats, spinach, and legumes help prevent anemia, and fatty fish and fortified foods provide vitamin D.

B vitamins are found in whole grains, eggs, and leafy greens, while vitamin C is abundant in citrus fruits, bell peppers, and strawberries. The worst way to manage deficiencies is relying solely on processed and fast foods, which often lack essential nutrients and contribute to poor health. Avoiding nutrient-poor diets and focusing on diverse, whole-food nutrition ensures that the body receives the vitamins and minerals needed for optimal function and long-term well-being.

Importance of Hydration

Hydration is essential for overall health, as water plays a critical role in nearly every bodily function, including temperature regulation, digestion, circulation, and nutrient absorption. The human body is composed of about 60% water, making proper hydration vital for maintaining energy levels, cognitive function, and organ health. The positive effects of staying well-hydrated include improved brain function, enhanced physical performance, better digestion, detoxification, and healthier skin.

Proper hydration helps flush out toxins, prevents kidney stones, supports joint lubrication, and regulates body temperature. It also aids in weight management by promoting satiety and preventing overeating, as thirst is often mistaken for hunger. However, dehydration can have negative effects, leading to fatigue, headaches, dizziness, poor concentration, constipation, and an increased risk of kidney stones and urinary tract infections.

Severe dehydration can cause heatstroke, low blood pressure, and, in extreme cases, organ failure. Overhydration, though rare, can also be harmful, leading to water intoxication (hyponatremia), where excess water dilutes essential electrolytes such as sodium, causing swelling in the brain and other serious health issues. The best sources of hydration are pure water, herbal teas, coconut water, and water-rich foods like cucumbers, watermelon, oranges, and celery. These provide hydration while also offering additional nutrients and electrolytes.

The worst sources of hydration include sugary sodas, excessive caffeine, and alcoholic beverages, as they can contribute to dehydration, blood sugar imbalances, and other health problems. Maintaining proper hydration by drinking enough water daily, based on individual needs and activity levels, ensures optimal body function, energy levels, and overall well-being.

The Hidden Salt in Bottled Water: Why You Need to Pay Attention

When we think about hydration, we often assume that all bottled water is the same: clear, refreshing, and healthy. But what many people don't realize is that **some bottled waters contain added salts**, and drinking these types of water regularly can pose hidden health risks. This is an important subject that's often overlooked, but understanding what's in your water is just as vital as paying attention to what's on your plate.

Recognizing Salts in Bottled Water

Not all bottled waters are created equal. Some types of bottled water, particularly **mineral water** or **alkaline water**, can contain varying levels of **salts** or **sodium**. While salts naturally occur in some water sources, they can also be added during the bottling process. This is often done to enhance the flavor or increase the mineral content. To **recognize water with added salts**, you need to read the label. Check for terms like:

- **Sodium** (salt is made up of sodium and chloride)
- **Mineral content** or **electrolytes**
- **Sodium bicarbonate** or **calcium salts**

Even if the label simply says "mineral water," it can still contain sodium or other salts that may not be immediately obvious. Look at the **mineral content section** of the label to identify how much sodium or salt is in the water.

Why It's Dangerous to Drink Water with Added Salts

While your body does need some sodium for various functions (like regulating blood pressure and maintaining fluid balance), **too much sodium can be harmful**, especially when it's consumed through drinking water over time. High sodium intake is linked to a variety of health problems, including:

- **High blood pressure (hypertension):** Sodium increases the volume of blood in your bloodstream, which can raise blood pressure, putting strain on your heart and arteries.
- **Kidney damage:** Your kidneys work hard to filter excess sodium from your blood, and over time, high sodium levels can strain your kidneys, potentially leading to kidney disease.
- **Dehydration:** Ironically, drinking water with a high salt content can actually contribute to dehydration. Sodium pulls water from your cells and into your bloodstream, which can leave you feeling thirsty even after drinking.
- **Bloating and swelling:** Consuming too much salt causes your body to retain water, which can lead to bloating and swelling, particularly in your hands, feet, and face.

The Importance of Drinking Spring Water

Now, contrast that with **spring water**, which is naturally filtered through rocks and soil, often containing a balance of **essential minerals** that are beneficial to your health, without the harmful added salts. **Spring water** is a natural, unprocessed option that can help keep your body hydrated and balanced without the risk of excess sodium intake.

Spring water is often richer in minerals like calcium, magnesium, and potassium, which are essential for muscle function, bone health, and maintaining fluid balance in the body. These minerals, in their natural form, contribute to a more balanced and healthier hydration source.

How Spring Water Makes Me Feel Healthier

Since I made the conscious decision to switch from bottled water with added salts to drinking **pure spring water**, I've noticed a significant improvement in how I feel. Initially, I didn't realize how much excess sodium was affecting my energy levels, bloating, and overall health. I used to feel sluggish after drinking certain bottled waters, but when I switched to spring water, I noticed a clearer, more energized state. Drinking **pure spring water** has helped:

- **Reduce bloating and water retention:** Since I stopped drinking water with added salts, I've noticed less puffiness in my face and body.

- **Increase my energy:** Without excess sodium pulling water from my cells, I feel more hydrated, which leads to more sustained energy throughout the day.
- **Better digestion:** The natural balance of minerals in spring water seems to support better digestion and overall gut health.
- **Enhanced mental clarity:** Hydration with mineral-rich spring water has contributed to better mental focus and clarity, helping me feel more present and sharp.

Switching to spring water has made a world of difference in how my body feels and functions. **It's a simple change**, but the effects have been noticeable in my day-to-day life.

Conclusion: Choose Wisely

Water is essential to life, but not all water is created equally. When choosing bottled water, it's important to be mindful of its contents. While some bottled waters contain added salts that can be harmful over time, others, like **pure spring water,** offer a healthier alternative, with natural minerals that support your body's hydration needs without the added risks of excess sodium.

Your body deserves the best, and drinking **spring water** is a simple and effective way to ensure you're hydrating the right way. By paying attention to the labels and choosing water that nourishes rather than harms, you can significantly improve your overall health and feel better than ever. Start drinking the right kind of water today, and see how it transforms your health from the inside out.

How Much Water Do You Need?

A general guideline is to drink at least 8 cups (2 liters) of water per day, but individual needs vary based on factors such as age, gender, activity level, and climate. Listening to your body's thirst signals and consuming water-rich foods like fruits and vegetables can help maintain proper hydration.

Understanding Metabolism & Basal Metabolic Rate (BMR)

Basal Metabolic Rate (BMR) is the amount of energy your body needs to maintain basic functions while at rest. BMR accounts for about 60-75% of your total daily energy expenditure. It's influenced by factors like age, sex, weight, height, and body composition. BMR calculations provide a baseline for estimating how many calories your body requires daily just to sustain vital physiological processes, such as breathing, circulation, and cell function, without considering physical activity or digestion.

Understanding your BMR is essential for tailoring your nutrition and fitness plans to achieve weight management goals. By knowing your BMR, you can calculate your Total Daily Energy Expenditure (TDEE), which includes calories burned through daily activities and exercise. This knowledge helps you create a calorie deficit for weight loss or a surplus for muscle gain, based on your specific goals and metabolic needs.

Factors like muscle mass significantly influence BMR; muscle tissue burns more calories than fat tissue, even at rest. Age-related decreases in BMR can occur due to reductions in muscle mass and hormonal changes. Practical applications of BMR calculations involve using formulas or specialized equipment to estimate metabolic rates accurately, guiding adjustments in dietary intake and physical activity levels to support overall health and fitness goals effectively.

Total Daily Energy Expenditure (TDEE)

Understanding Total Daily Energy Expenditure (TDEE) has been a game-changer for me in managing my weight and health. TDEE represents the total number of calories I need to maintain my current weight, factoring in all my daily activities and bodily functions. It's made up of Basal Metabolic Rate (BMR), the Thermic Effect of Food (TEF), calories burned through physical activity, and the Thermic Effect of Activity (TEA). By calculating my BMR using the Harris-Benedict or Mifflin-St Jeor equations and then adjusting for my activity level, I get a clear picture of my TDEE.

Knowing my TDEE has allowed me to tailor my diet and exercise plans effectively. To maintain my weight, I aim to consume calories equal to my TDEE. When I want to lose weight, I create a calorie deficit by eating fewer calories than my TDEE, usually by cutting about 500 calories per day. On the other hand, if I want to gain weight, I create a calorie surplus by consuming 250-500 more calories daily than my TDEE. Factors like age, sex, body composition, genetics, and lifestyle have all influenced my TDEE, so I adjust my approach accordingly.

Regularly tracking my progress and tweaking my calorie intake based on my activity levels and goals has been crucial. I've found that using apps and wearable devices to estimate my TDEE and track my calorie intake and expenditure makes it much easier to stay on track. Additionally, consulting with dietitians and fitness trainers has provided me with personalized guidance, ensuring that my weight-management strategies are both effective and sustainable. Understanding and utilizing TDEE has empowered me to take control of my health and achieve my fitness goals.

Calculating Your Caloric Needs

To create a caloric deficit, you need to know your TDEE. Several online calculators can help you estimate your TDEE based on factors such as age, gender, weight, height, and activity level. Once you know your TDEE, you can create a caloric deficit by consuming fewer calories or increasing your physical activity.

Calculating my calorie needs has been essential in managing my weight effectively. I started by determining my Basal Metabolic Rate (BMR), which is the number of calories my body needs at rest to maintain basic functions. Using formulas like the Harris-Benedict or Mifflin-St Jeor Equation, which consider factors such as age, sex, weight, and height, I was able to calculate my BMR accurately.

Next, I figured out my activity level by considering my daily routines and exercise habits. By multiplying my BMR by an activity level factor from sedentary (BMR × 1.2) to super active (BMR × 1.9) I calculated my Total Daily Energy Expenditure (TDEE). For instance, as a moderately active 40-year-old man weighing 265 pounds, my TDEE came out to approximately 3394 calories per day.

With my TDEE in hand, I tailored my calorie intake to meet my weight goals. To lose weight, I created a calorie deficit by consuming fewer calories than my TDEE, reducing my daily intake by about 1500 calories to aim for a weekly weight loss of around 1.5 kg (3 pounds). Alternatively, if you want to increase your weight, increase your intake by 250-500 calories above your TDEE; consult a licensed professional for healthy goals to strive for. Understanding my calorie needs has empowered me to make informed decisions about my diet and exercise, helping me achieve and maintain my desired weight.

The Role of Hormones in Weight Regulation

Insulin

Insulin is a hormone produced by the pancreas that helps regulate blood sugar levels. It allows your cells to take in glucose from the bloodstream and use it for energy. When you consume carbohydrates, your blood sugar levels rise, prompting the release of insulin. Managing insulin levels through balanced eating and regular physical activity is crucial for weight loss.

Leptin

Leptin is a hormone produced by fat cells that signals to your brain when you're full. It helps regulate energy balance and suppresses appetite. However, in cases of obesity, leptin resistance can occur, meaning the brain doesn't respond to leptin signals effectively, leading to overeating. Understanding leptin's role can help you make better dietary choices.

Ghrelin

Ghrelin, known as the "hunger hormone," is produced in the stomach and stimulates appetite. Ghrelin levels increase before meals and decrease after eating. Managing ghrelin levels through regular meals, adequate sleep, and stress reduction can help control hunger and support weight loss.

Understanding metabolism has been crucial for managing my health and fitness. Metabolism encompasses all the processes that convert the food I eat into energy for my body's functions. It includes both breaking down molecules to release energy (catabolism) and using energy to build cellular components (anabolism). Knowing how my metabolism works helps me make better decisions about my diet, exercise, and overall lifestyle.

Physical activity significantly impacts my metabolism. The more active I am, the more calories I burn. Whether it's walking, typing, exercising, or doing manual labor, physical activities increase my metabolic rate. High-intensity exercises, like weight training and high-intensity interval training (HIIT), are particularly effective because they keep my metabolism elevated even after I finish working out.

The thermic effect of food (TEF) is another component of metabolism that I've learned to consider. TEF is the energy required to digest, absorb, and process the nutrients from the food I eat. It accounts for about 10% of my total daily energy expenditure.

I've found that different macronutrients have different thermic effects: protein has the highest, followed by carbohydrates and fats. This insight has encouraged me to include more protein in my diet to boost my metabolism.

Metabolic processes like catabolism and anabolism are fascinating. Catabolism involves breaking down molecules to produce energy, such as through glycolysis and the Krebs cycle. Anabolism, on the other hand, uses this energy to build essential molecules like proteins and fatty acids. Understanding these processes has given me a deeper appreciation of how my body uses the food I eat.

Several factors affect my metabolism beyond just diet and exercise. Genetics play a significant role, as my metabolic rate can be partly inherited. Muscle mass is another critical factor more muscle increases my BMR, since muscle tissue requires more energy to maintain than fat tissue. Hormones, particularly thyroid hormones and insulin, also regulate my metabolism.

I've found that lifestyle choices, such as sleep and hydration, profoundly impact my metabolism. Poor sleep disrupts the hormones that regulate hunger and energy expenditure, often leading to weight gain. Staying hydrated is essential because water is involved in numerous metabolic processes. Ensuring that I get enough rest and drink plenty of water helps keep my metabolism functioning optimally.

To boost my metabolism, I focus on building muscle through strength training, staying active, eating protein-rich foods, staying hydrated, getting adequate sleep, and eating smaller, more frequent meals. These strategies help keep my metabolism active and efficient, supporting my overall health and fitness goals. Understanding my metabolism has empowered me to make informed decisions and maintain a healthier lifestyle. Be sure to consult a licensed professional to help you understand your individual health needs.

Chapter 3

Know Your Body

The Importance of Knowing Your Body: Listening to What It's Telling You

One of the most valuable lessons I've learned on my health journey is the importance of truly knowing your body, not just in terms of appearance or how much weight you've gained or lost, but by paying close attention to the subtle signals and functions your body is constantly sending you. Your body communicates with you every day, and understanding those messages is key to taking control of your health.

For many years, I ignored the warning signs, brushing off fatigue, digestive issues, and irritability as something "normal" or "temporary." But what I learned through my journey is that our bodies are incredibly wise, and when something is off, it's often a reflection of what's happening inside. If we ignore those signals for too long, they can escalate into bigger health problems.

Understanding Your Energy Levels

One of the most basic and important functions of your body is energy. Your energy level is one of the first signs that can indicate whether something is off. Fatigue isn't something you should just accept as part of life, especially if it becomes constant or excessive. When you're well-rested and nourished, your energy should feel balanced throughout the day, with manageable ups and downs. However, if you're feeling tired all the time, it could be a sign of nutrient deficiencies, poor sleep patterns, or even underlying health issues like thyroid problems or anemia.

Pay attention to your energy levels. If you're feeling exhausted even after getting a full night's sleep, or if you have bursts of energy followed by sharp crashes, these are signs that your body is trying to tell you something. Listen to it, because your body functions better when it's properly fueled.

The Role of Digestion and Gut Health

Another major area where you need to tune in is your digestive system. Digestion is central to your overall health. If you're feeling bloated, constipated, or suffering from stomach aches regularly, those aren't just discomforts you have to live with; they're red flags. Your digestive system can give you direct insight into what's going on in your body.

Gut health plays a massive role in how you absorb nutrients, maintain your immune system, and even your mood. In fact, the gut is sometimes referred to as the "second brain" because of its profound effect on mental health. Regular issues with digestion could signal imbalances, food sensitivities, or even an inflammatory response to the foods you're eating.

Pay attention to how your body responds to food. If certain foods make you feel sluggish, bloated, or irritable, it's important to consider that your body may be telling you something about how it processes those foods. Keeping track of your meals and how you feel afterward can help you identify patterns and make necessary changes.

Skin as a Reflection of Your Inner Health

The condition of your skin is another external indicator of your internal health. Skin problems like acne, eczema, or dryness can be symptoms of nutritional deficiencies, dehydration, or hormonal imbalances. If your skin is constantly breaking out, dry, or irritated, it's not just about cosmetic issues; it could be a signal that your body needs more hydration, better nutrition, or a deeper look at hormone levels.

Know your skin. Take note of any changes in texture, breakouts, rashes, or discoloration, and try to connect them with your diet, stress levels, or hydration habits. Your skin is a reflection of your overall health, and paying attention to it can help you make improvements to your internal wellness.

Mental and Emotional Signals

Your body also sends out signals through your emotions and mental clarity. If you're feeling stressed, anxious, or overwhelmed, your body is reacting to external pressures. However, emotional distress can also be linked to physical health issues. For example, prolonged stress can lead to chronic inflammation, digestive issues, or even high blood pressure.

Tune in to your mental state. If you're feeling mentally foggy or having difficulty focusing, it could be a sign that your body is under stress, lacks nutrients, or isn't getting enough rest. Anxiety or irritability can also be linked to blood sugar imbalances or dehydration. Understanding the connection between your physical state and mental health will help you make better choices for both.

Sleep and Rest: The Body's Repair System

Sleep is one of the most vital processes that your body uses to recharge, repair, and restore balance. If you're having trouble falling asleep, staying asleep, or waking up feeling unrested, your body is telling you that something's wrong. Poor sleep is often associated with a poor diet, high levels of stress, or an underlying medical condition.

Observe your sleep patterns. Your body's ability to rest and recover affects everything from your energy levels to your emotional health. If you're waking up tired every day or having trouble getting deep sleep, it may be time to reassess your habits, environment, or consult a doctor for potential sleep disorders.

The Power of Hydration

One of the most overlooked yet essential functions of the body is hydration. Often, we forget that our bodies are made up of about 60% water, and everything from digestion to circulation depends on staying hydrated. Dehydration can lead to headaches, fatigue, dry skin, and constipation, just to name a few.

Pay attention to your thirst. If you're not thirsty but still experience these symptoms, you may not be getting enough water or the right balance of electrolytes. Keep track of your hydration levels throughout the day and aim to drink at least eight cups of water, or more if you're physically active or live in a hot climate. I can't stress this enough. Knowing and doing this will keep you out of the hospital and safe.

Respect and Respond to Your Body

Knowing your body is an ongoing process. It's about understanding how your body functions, recognizing when something feels off, and having the awareness to take action. Your body will always give you clues; it's just a matter of paying attention. Whether it's energy levels, digestion, skin health, mental clarity, or sleep, each of these functions plays a crucial role in your overall well-being.

Don't wait until your body is in crisis to start listening. Take the time to tune in to your body's signals today. Listen to your body's needs, respond to them, and treat it with the respect it deserves. By doing so, you'll empower yourself to make healthier decisions, improve your quality of life, and maintain a balanced, thriving body.

Body Mass Index (BMI)

BMI, or Body Mass Index, is a measure used to evaluate body weight relative to height. It's calculated by dividing weight in kilograms by height in meters squared, or, for those using pounds and inches, by multiplying weight in pounds by 703 and dividing by height in inches squared. The resulting number categorizes individuals into underweight, normal weight, overweight, or obese categories. For me, BMI has been a straightforward way to gauge my weight status and potential health risks associated with it.

While BMI provides a quick snapshot of body fat based on weight and height, it has its limitations. It doesn't distinguish between muscle mass and fat mass, so individuals with higher muscle may register as overweight or obese despite being healthy. Despite its simplicity, I find it helpful as a starting point for understanding my health and discussing weight management with my healthcare provider.

Body Composition

Body composition refers to the proportion of fat and lean mass (muscles, bones, water) in your body. Methods to measure body composition include skin-fold measurements, bioelectrical impedance analysis (BIA), dual-energy X-ray absorptiometry (DXA), and hydrostatic weighing. Understanding your body composition provides a more comprehensive picture of your health than BMI alone.

Health Conditions

Certain health conditions can affect weight loss and require special consideration. Conditions such as hypothyroidism, polycystic ovary syndrome (PCOS), and insulin resistance can impact metabolism and weight regulation. Consulting with a healthcare provider can help identify any underlying conditions and develop a tailored weight-loss plan.

Navigating weight loss with health conditions has been a challenging yet enlightening journey for me. Conditions like hypothyroidism have significantly impacted my metabolism, making it difficult to shed excess weight despite my efforts. The sluggish thyroid function has slowed down calorie burning, requiring a more vigilant approach to diet and exercise to maintain a healthy weight.

I've also grappled with the effects of medications prescribed for mental health conditions, which have occasionally caused weight gain as a side effect. Managing depression and anxiety has been crucial, as these conditions influence my appetite and eating habits, sometimes making it harder to stick to healthy eating patterns. The interplay of these factors has taught me the importance of a holistic approach to weight management that considers both physical health conditions and mental well-being.

Furthermore, chronic stress has played a role in my weight journey, elevating cortisol levels and triggering cravings that can derail my efforts. Learning effective stress management techniques has been pivotal in maintaining a balanced approach to weight loss. Through personalized strategies developed with healthcare professionals, including medication adjustments and targeted dietary plans, I've been able to navigate these challenges and work toward achieving a sustainable, healthy weight.

Managing weight loss with various health conditions requires a calculated approach that considers how each condition impacts metabolism, hormone regulation, and overall health. Conditions like type 2 diabetes and heart disease can affect weight through factors such as insulin resistance, medication side effects, and limitations in physical activity. Hormonal imbalances, including those related to thyroid disorders or adrenal gland dysfunction, can also complicate weight management by altering metabolic processes and energy balance.

Additionally, chronic pain conditions like osteoarthritis or fibromyalgia, as well as gastrointestinal disorders and sleep apnea, present further challenges. These conditions may limit mobility, affect nutrient absorption, disrupt sleep patterns, or lead to changes in appetite and metabolism. Successfully navigating weight loss in the presence of these conditions often requires a tailored approach that integrates medical management, dietary modifications, physical activity adjustments, and psychological support to address both the physical and emotional aspects of health.

Incorporating personalized strategies developed with healthcare professionals is crucial for individuals facing these challenges, ensuring a comprehensive plan that promotes sustainable weight loss and enhances overall well-being. Setting SMART goals can help you stay focused and motivated. For example, instead of setting a vague goal like "lose weight," set a specific goal such as "lose 10 pounds in 3 months by exercising 30 minutes a day and reducing daily calorie intake by 500 calories." "

Setting SMART goals involves creating clear and specific objectives that are measurable, achievable, relevant, and time-bound. For me, this approach has been invaluable in achieving meaningful outcomes. By defining exactly what I want to accomplish and why it matters to me, I gain clarity and motivation to pursue my goals effectively. Setting measurable criteria allows me to track progress and celebrate milestones along the way, reinforcing my commitment and boosting my confidence.

Ensuring that my goals are achievable and realistic helps me stay grounded in what is feasible given my current resources and circumstances. Aligning each goal with my long-term aspirations ensures that my efforts are meaningful and contribute positively to my overall journey. Establishing clear deadlines keeps me accountable and focused, providing a sense of urgency that drives consistent action toward achieving my desired outcomes. Embracing the SMART framework has empowered me to set goals that are not only challenging but also within reach, fostering continuous growth and success in various areas of my life.

Short-term and Long-term Goals

Breaking down your overall weight loss goal into short-term and long-term goals can make the process more manageable. Short-term goals might include weekly or monthly targets, while long-term goals focus on overall weight loss and health improvements over several months or a year.

To begin, make your goal specific by clearly defining what you want to achieve, such as losing 20 pounds or reducing body fat by 5%. Instead of a vague goal like "I want to lose weight," a specific goal would be, "I want to lose 15 pounds by following a balanced diet and exercising five days a week." "

Next, ensure your goal is measurable by setting benchmarks to track progress. This could include weighing yourself weekly, measuring inches lost, or tracking calorie intake and burned calories through an app. An achievable goal is one that is realistic based on your current lifestyle, health, and resources.

Losing 1-2 pounds per week is a healthy and sustainable target rather than aiming for drastic weight loss in a short period, which can be unhealthy and difficult to maintain. Your goal should also be relevant, meaning it aligns with your personal motivations, whether it's improving overall health, boosting confidence, or preparing for an event. Finally, your goal must be time-bound, meaning it has a clear deadline to maintain focus and motivation.

Embracing a Long-term Perspective

Understanding that weight loss is a marathon, not a sprint, is crucial. Rapid weight loss is often unsustainable and can lead to health issues. Focus on making gradual changes that you can maintain in the long term. Developing patience while losing weight has been a transformative journey for me. I've learned firsthand the importance of setting realistic goals and celebrating even the smallest achievements along the way. By focusing on sustainable habits rather than quick fixes, such as adopting a balanced diet and staying physically active, I've cultivated patience in knowing that meaningful changes take time.

Practicing mindfulness techniques, such as meditation and deep breathing, has been instrumental in managing my impatience and staying committed to my goals. Tracking my progress through a journal has allowed me to see how far I've come and stay motivated despite occasional setbacks. The support of my friends and family has been invaluable, providing encouragement and accountability when I needed it most. Learning from setbacks has taught me resilience and reinforced my dedication to achieving a healthier lifestyle, one step at a time.

Acknowledging and celebrating small victories along the way can boost your motivation and confidence. Whether it's losing a few pounds, fitting into a smaller clothing size, or improving your fitness level, recognizing these achievements helps reinforce your commitment to your goals.

Chapter 4

Stress Management Is Weight Management

It is very important to know your mind even more than you know your body. Do you know the why behind your eating habits? One of the things I found that caused me to eat the most was stress. When I was emotional about something, I relieved myself with food. Sometimes food can be the easiest and most satisfying way to create a feeling of comfort; after all, they don't call it "comfort food" for nothing. I sought professional help, and my stress levels changed; then I noticed I was able to lose weight at the same pace as I once did, and that's when I began to learn.

Stress management plays a crucial role in weight loss, as chronic stress can disrupt metabolism, increase fat storage, and trigger unhealthy eating habits. When the body experiences stress, it activates the hypothalamic-pituitary-adrenal (HPA) axis, leading to the release of cortisol, a hormone that, when elevated for prolonged periods, contributes to weight gain, particularly around the abdomen.

Managing stress effectively has numerous benefits for weight loss, including reducing emotional eating, balancing hormones, improving sleep quality, boosting energy levels, and enhancing digestion. Lower cortisol levels make it easier to regulate appetite, prevent binge eating, and support muscle recovery, all of which contribute to a more efficient metabolism and sustainable weight loss.

On the other hand, uncontrolled stress can sabotage weight loss efforts by increasing cravings for high-calorie, sugary, and fatty foods. It also slows down metabolism, causes insulin resistance, and disrupts sleep patterns, leading to poor food choices and increased hunger. Additionally, high cortisol levels can interfere with muscle growth and recovery, making it harder to build lean muscle, which is essential for burning fat. Poor stress management often leads to emotional eating, skipping meals, excessive caffeine or alcohol consumption, and a sedentary lifestyle, all of which make it more difficult to achieve and maintain a healthy weight.

Implementing effective stress management strategies is essential for optimizing weight loss. Mindfulness techniques, such as meditation, deep breathing, journaling, and practicing gratitude, help lower cortisol levels and improve emotional regulation. Engaging in physical activity, such as cardio, strength training, yoga, or outdoor activities, not only burns calories but also releases endorphins that counteract stress.

Quality sleep is another critical factor, as poor sleep increases hunger hormones and cravings. A consistent sleep routine, limiting screen time before bed, and avoiding caffeine late in the day can significantly improve sleep quality. Nutrition also plays a vital role in stress management: eating a balanced diet with whole foods, lean proteins, healthy fats, and fiber-rich carbohydrates helps regulate blood sugar levels and prevents stress-induced cravings. Staying hydrated, consuming magnesium-rich foods, and avoiding processed and sugary foods further support stress reduction.

Social support and emotional well-being are equally important in managing stress for weight loss. Spending time with loved ones, joining a wellness or weight loss community, and seeking professional guidance through therapy or coaching can provide motivation and accountability. Effective time management, setting boundaries, and prioritizing self-care reduce feelings of overwhelm, preventing stress from interfering with healthy habits. Additionally, limiting stimulants like caffeine and alcohol, which can heighten stress responses, and opting for calming herbal teas can further aid relaxation.

Avoiding negative stress management habits is just as crucial as implementing positive strategies. Emotional eating, skipping meals, overtraining, excessive alcohol consumption, and neglecting sleep can all worsen stress and hinder weight loss progress. Instead, taking a holistic approach that balances mental, emotional, and physical health is key to long-term success. By integrating mindfulness, movement, proper nutrition, rest, and social support, individuals can effectively manage stress, enhance metabolism, and achieve sustainable weight loss while improving overall well-being.

Engaging in specific exercises can effectively reduce stress by releasing endorphins, lowering cortisol levels, and improving overall mental well-being. Here are some of the best exercises for stress relief:

Walking (Especially in Nature) – A simple, low-impact way to reduce stress while improving mood and cardiovascular health. Walking in green spaces (forest bathing) has been shown to lower cortisol levels significantly. Running or Jogging – Releases endorphins, improves circulation, and helps clear the mind from anxious thoughts. Cycling – Whether outdoors or on a stationary bike, cycling provides a rhythmic movement that promotes relaxation and stress relief. Dancing – A fun way to relieve stress while improving coordination and cardiovascular health. Dancing to music also stimulates positive emotions. Jump Rope – A quick, high-intensity exercise that improves cardiovascular health and reduces tension.

Weightlifting – Lifting weights or using resistance bands helps focus the mind, reduces tension, and builds confidence. Body-weight Exercises (Push-Ups, Squats, Planks, Lunges) – Engaging multiple muscle groups helps release endorphins and provides a sense of accomplishment. Yoga – Combines movement, breathing, and mindfulness to promote relaxation, improve flexibility, and reduce anxiety. Styles such as Hatha and Yin yoga are particularly effective for stress relief.

Tai Chi – A slow, meditative martial art that focuses on controlled movements and breathing to calm the nervous system. Pilates – Strengthens core muscles while promoting controlled breathing and body awareness, reducing mental and physical stress.

Deep Breathing Exercises – Techniques such as the 4-7-8 breathing method (inhale for 4 seconds, hold for 7, exhale for 8) or box breathing help lower heart rate and induce relaxation. Progressive Muscle Relaxation (PMR) – Involves tensing and relaxing muscle groups to relieve tension and calm the body.

Hiking – Being in nature combined with physical movement reduces stress and enhances mental clarity. Swimming – The rhythmic breathing and resistance of water create a calming effect, easing tension and reducing anxiety. Kayaking or Paddleboarding – Engages the upper body while promoting relaxation and a connection with nature. Gardening – Though not a high-intensity workout, gardening involves physical movement, deep breathing, and exposure to nature, all of which help reduce stress.

Short Bursts of High-Energy Movements (Jump Squats, Burpees, Sprints) – HIIT workouts help burn off excess energy and release endorphins while improving cardiovascular fitness. Foam Rolling (Myofascial Release) – Helps release tension in tight muscles, improve blood circulation, and aid in relaxation. Static & Dynamic Stretching – Improves flexibility, reduces muscle stiffness, and encourages deep breathing for relaxation. Incorporating any of these exercises into your routine can significantly reduce stress, improve mood, and enhance overall well-being. While doing it on your own is optional, the benefits of getting help can be far greater than going it alone.

Seeking professional help to deal with stress and trauma was one of the best decisions I ever made for my weight loss journey. For years, I struggled with emotional eating, inconsistent motivation, and feeling stuck in a cycle of unhealthy habits. No matter how hard I tried to control my diet and exercise, stress and unresolved trauma always pulled me back into old patterns.

It wasn't until I worked with a therapist that I realized my weight issues weren't just about food and exercise; they were deeply connected to my emotions, past experiences, and the way I coped with stress. Therapy helped me recognize my triggers, break free from self-sabotaging behaviors, and develop healthier coping mechanisms that didn't involve food.

Through counseling, I learned how to manage anxiety, reframe negative thoughts, and set realistic goals without being too hard on myself. My therapist also helped me uncover the root causes of my stress, whether they stemmed from childhood experiences, daily pressures, or deep-seated fears. Instead of turning to comfort food when I felt overwhelmed, I learned mindful techniques like deep breathing, journaling, and self-compassion. Professional help gave me the tools to heal, making weight loss feel less like a battle and more like a natural byproduct of taking care of myself.

Working with a nutritionist also played a huge role in my transformation. I happen to be a chef, so it was easy for me to cook healthy meals. I used to think weight loss was just about cutting calories, instead of understanding the importance of nourishing my body rather than depriving it. I learned how certain foods could either fuel stress or help me manage it, and that eating well was about balance, not restriction.

I found exercises that reduced my stress and improved my mental health. Most importantly, professional help reminded me that I didn't have to do it alone. I had spent so much time believing that weight loss was just about willpower, but I learned that emotional healing is just as important as physical effort. Therapy, coaching, and support groups gave me the accountability, encouragement, and structured strategies I needed to truly transform. My journey wasn't just about losing weight; it was about healing from the inside out. Now, I don't just look better; I feel stronger, more in control, and finally at peace with my body and mind.

Chapter 5

Building A Healthy Diet

""""The Importance of Building a Healthy Diet: Nourishing Your Body from the Inside Out

Building a healthy diet isn't just about choosing the right foods; it's about making conscious decisions that support your body's long-term health, energy levels, and overall well-being. Many of us know that what we eat plays a role in how we feel, but a truly healthy diet goes beyond temporary solutions. It's about creating a balanced, sustainable way of eating that nourishes your body and helps you thrive, both physically and mentally.

Why Building a Healthy Diet Matters

When we think about food, it's easy to focus on weight loss, dieting, or quick fixes. But the truth is that what we choose to fuel our bodies with has a lasting impact on everything from our energy levels to our immune system. Here's why building a healthy diet should be one of your top priorities:

1. Fuels Your Energy and Productivity

Your body relies on the food you eat for energy. When you make healthy choices, you're giving your body the nutrients it needs to perform at its best. Think of your body like a car: if you put low-quality fuel into it, it won't run efficiently, and eventually, it will break down. Eating a balanced diet, rich in whole foods like fruits, vegetables, lean proteins, and healthy fats, provides consistent, long-lasting energy to power through your day. On the other hand, a poor diet filled with processed foods and excessive sugar can lead to energy crashes, brain fog, and a lack of focus, making it difficult to stay productive or motivated. Building a healthy diet ensures your body is properly fueled, which helps you maintain consistent energy levels throughout the day.

2. Strengthens Your Immune System

Your immune system is your body's first line of defense against infections and diseases. A healthy diet provides the vitamins, minerals, and antioxidants that your immune system needs to fight off harmful pathogens. Nutrients like vitamin C, zinc, vitamin D, and selenium are crucial for immune function. Eating a variety of colorful fruits and vegetables, whole grains, and lean proteins helps ensure that you're getting a wide range of these essential nutrients.

""""When you fuel your body with nutrient-dense foods, you give your immune system the best chance of performing at its best, reducing your risk of chronic illnesses and helping you recover faster when you do get sick.

3. Promotes Healthy Digestion

A balanced diet filled with fiber-rich foods, such as fruits, vegetables, whole grains, and legumes, supports a healthy digestive system. Fiber helps keep your digestive tract functioning properly by promoting regular bowel movements, preventing constipation, and feeding beneficial gut bacteria. Gut health is closely linked to overall well-being, influencing everything from mental health to immune function.

If your diet lacks fiber, you may experience digestive discomfort, bloating, or irregularity. Building a healthy diet that includes a variety of fiber-rich foods helps keep your digestion on track and contributes to better gut health overall.

4. Supports Healthy Weight Management

One of the most significant reasons to build a healthy diet is to maintain a healthy weight. When your body gets the right balance of nutrients, you're less likely to experience cravings, overeating, or emotional eating. A healthy diet that includes a balance of protein, healthy fats, and complex carbohydrates can help you feel fuller for longer, making it easier to manage portion sizes and avoid unhealthy snacking. Moreover, a well-rounded diet, rather than focusing on restrictive eating, helps your metabolism function optimally and supports fat loss while preserving lean muscle mass. Building a healthy diet is about finding balance, not deprivation. It helps you create sustainable habits that lead to long-term success, rather than quick fixes that don't last.

5. Improves Mental Clarity and Emotional Well-being

What you eat not only affects your body but also your mind. A diet rich in omega-3 fatty acids, antioxidants, vitamins, and minerals plays a crucial role in cognitive function, mood regulation, and mental clarity.""" Foods like fatty fish (salmon, mackerel), leafy greens, berries, and nuts provide the brain with the nutrients it needs to function at its best, helping improve focus, memory, and mood.

On the other hand, diets high in processed sugars, unhealthy fats, and refined carbs have been linked to mood swings, irritability, and even conditions like depression and anxiety. Building a healthy diet with a focus on nourishing, whole foods helps support mental health, keeps your mood stable, and improves overall emotional well-being.

6. Reduces the risk of chronic diseases

Perhaps the most important reason to build a healthy diet is to reduce the risk of chronic disease. A well-balanced diet can prevent and even reverse many chronic conditions, such as heart disease, type 2 diabetes, and hypertension. By focusing on whole, nutrient-dense foods and avoiding processed foods high in added sugars, unhealthy fats, and sodium, you can significantly reduce your risk of developing these conditions. The impact of a healthy diet on long-term health cannot be overstated. Consuming nutrient-rich foods lowers inflammation, improves heart health, stabilizes blood sugar levels, and promotes better cholesterol levels, all of which contribute to a longer, healthier life.

Meal Planning and Preparation

Components of a Balanced Meal

A balanced meal includes a mix of macronutrients (proteins, carbohydrates, and fats) and micronutrients (vitamins and minerals). Aim to fill half your plate with vegetables and fruits, a quarter with lean proteins, and a quarter with whole grains, complemented by a small amount of healthy fats.

Portion Control

Portion control is key to maintaining a healthy diet and weight effectively. It involves understanding the appropriate amount of food to consume at each meal, which may differ from standard serving sizes. Practical tools like using your hand as a guide for protein, vegetables, carbohydrates, and fats, or using measuring cups and spoons, help ensure you're not overeating. The plate method, dividing your plate into portions for vegetables or fruits, lean protein, and whole grains or starchy foods, provides a visual aid for balanced eating.

Mindful eating plays a crucial role in portion control, encouraging awareness of hunger and fullness cues to prevent overeating. By eating slowly and savoring meals, you can better gauge when you've had enough. Additionally, being mindful of portion sizes when dining out or snacking helps maintain overall calorie balance and supports healthy eating habits over time. Adjusting portion sizes based on individual needs and goals ensures that meals are both satisfying and nutritionally balanced.

Healthy Cooking Techniques

Opting for healthier cooking methods can reduce unnecessary calories and enhance nutrient retention. Techniques such as grilling, steaming, baking, and sautéing with minimal oil are preferable to frying or deep-frying.

Reducing Added Sugars and Salt

Limiting added sugars and salt in your diet is essential for preventing health issues like obesity, diabetes, and hypertension. Use natural sweeteners such as honey or maple syrup in moderation, and flavor your meals with herbs and spices instead of salt.

Low-Carb Diets

Low-carb diets are dietary approaches that significantly restrict carbohydrate intake while emphasizing a higher intake of protein and fat. Popular variations include the ketogenic diet (keto), which aims to induce ketosis by severely limiting carbs, and the low-carb, high-fat (LCHF) diet, which moderates carb intake while increasing healthy fats. These diets typically limit carbohydrates to 20-100 grams per day, promoting a shift in metabolism toward burning fat for energy rather than carbohydrates.

The primary benefits of low-carb diets include effective weight loss, often due to reduced calorie intake and initial water loss from glycogen stores. They can also improve blood sugar control, making them beneficial for managing diabetes and insulin resistance. Additionally, low-carb diets may lower triglyceride levels, increase HDL cholesterol (the "good" cholesterol), and improve markers of heart health. The higher protein and fat content of these diets may also enhance satiety, helping to control appetite and reduce overall calorie consumption.

However, there are considerations with low-carb diets. They can lead to initial side effects such as fatigue, headaches, and irritability, known as "keto flu," especially during the adjustment period. Long-term sustainability may be challenging for some individuals due to the restrictive nature of carbohydrate intake, which can limit food choices and social interactions. Nutrient deficiencies can also occur if not carefully planned, particularly in fiber, vitamins (especially B vitamins), and minerals like potassium and magnesium, typically found in higher-carbohydrate foods.

Personalizing a low-carb diet to individual needs and goals is crucial. This involves balancing carbohydrate intake with nutrient-dense foods like non-starchy vegetables, nuts, seeds, and low-carb fruits to ensure adequate nutrient intake. Regular monitoring of health markers and consulting with healthcare providers or dietitians can help optimize the benefits of a low-carb diet while addressing potential challenges and ensuring overall health and well-being.

Protein Diets

Protein diets, also known as high-protein diets, emphasize increasing protein intake while moderating carbohydrates and fats. They are popular for their role in muscle maintenance and growth, as proteins are essential for building and repairing tissues. Different types of protein diets exist, ranging from low-carb, high-protein approaches like the Atkins Diet to very high-protein regimens favored in bodybuilding circles. These diets often aim to promote weight loss, enhance muscle development, and improve metabolic health by prioritizing protein-rich foods.

The benefits of protein diets include improved muscle maintenance and growth, appetite control due to increased satiety from protein-rich foods, and potential enhancements in metabolic function, such as better insulin sensitivity and glucose regulation. These benefits can be particularly advantageous for athletes, individuals engaging in strength training, and those managing conditions like diabetes.

However, it's important to consider the overall nutrient balance when following protein diets. While protein is crucial, adequate intake of carbohydrates, fats, vitamins, and minerals is essential for overall health and well-being. Very high-protein diets, in particular, may pose risks to kidney health in individuals with existing kidney conditions due to increased strain on renal function.

Achieving a balanced protein intake involves incorporating a variety of protein sources into your diet, including both animal-based (meat, poultry, fish, dairy) and plant-based options (legumes, tofu, nuts, seeds). Consulting with a healthcare provider or a registered dietitian can help personalize a protein diet plan to meet individual nutritional needs and health goals, ensuring sustainable and effective results while minimizing potential risks. As with any dietary approach, the key to success lies in moderation, diversity, and personalized guidance to maintain optimal health outcomes.

Plant-Based Diets

Plant-based diets include vegetarian, vegan, and flexitarian diets. These diets focus on consuming plant-based foods such as fruits, vegetables, legumes, nuts, and seeds, with varying levels of animal-product consumption.

Health Benefits

A plant-based diet has become a cornerstone of my lifestyle, focusing on wholesome foods like fruits, vegetables, whole grains, nuts, and legumes while minimizing animal products. This dietary choice not only provides me with a wealth of vitamins, minerals, and antioxidants but also supports my overall health goals. I've noticed improvements in my heart health, with lower cholesterol levels and better blood pressure management, which aligns with my desire for a heart-healthy diet.

In addition to promoting weight management through natural calorie control and reduced saturated fats, my plant-based approach has heightened my awareness of nutrition. I prioritize fiber-rich foods that support digestive health, keeping me feeling energized and maintaining a healthy gut. However, I'm mindful of nutrient balance, ensuring adequate protein intake from sources like tofu, lentils, and nuts, while also incorporating supplements or fortified foods for essential nutrients like vitamin B12.

While navigating this dietary path, I'm conscious of sustainability and its environmental impact, appreciating how plant-based choices contribute to reducing my carbon footprint. Consult with a registered dietitian to fine-tune your plant-based diet to meet your individual nutritional needs and ensure long-term health and vitality. This personalized approach allows me to enjoy the benefits of a plant-based lifestyle while feeling confident in maintaining optimal health and well-being.

Intermittent Fasting

Intermittent fasting (IF) is an eating pattern that I find intriguing for its potential health benefits and flexibility. I've been exploring methods like the 16/8 approach, where I fast for 16 hours and eat within an 8-hour window daily, to manage my weight and improve metabolic health. I've also done the 5:2 diet, which involves regular eating for 5 days and reducing calorie intake to 500-600 calories on the remaining 2 days. These methods help me focus on reducing my overall calorie intake and enhancing fat burning during fasting periods.

I'm mindful of starting gradually and adjusting my eating patterns to suit my body's response and daily routine. Hydration during fasting periods is crucial for me, and ensuring balanced nutrition during eating windows remains a priority. Consulting with healthcare providers has been valuable in ensuring that I approach intermittent fasting safely, especially considering my individual health needs and goals. This personalized approach allows me to explore IF as a sustainable and beneficial part of my lifestyle.

Benefits and Considerations

Intermittent fasting can promote weight loss, improve metabolic health, and simplify meal planning. However, it may not be suitable for everyone, particularly those with a history of eating disorders or certain medical conditions. Consulting with a healthcare professional before starting intermittent fasting is recommended.

Chapter 6

My Favorite Lifestyle

Introduction to the Blood Type Diet

I want to share something that completely transformed my life: the *Eat Right 4 Your Type* diet. This approach, created by Dr. Peter D'Adamo, suggests that the foods we eat, the way we exercise, and even how we handle stress are influenced by our blood type. Sounds fascinating, right?

When I first heard about it, I was skeptical. But after following it, losing 350 pounds, I can tell you that this diet is worth exploring. Each blood type O, A, B, and AB has unique dietary recommendations designed to align with our genetic makeup. Let me break it down for you, sharing what works best for each type and how it could change your life, too.

Type O: The Hunter

Let's start with Type O, this is my blood type. Type O is considered the oldest blood type, linked to our hunter-gatherer ancestors. This explains why people with this blood type thrive on a high-protein diet. We're talking about lean meats like beef, lamb, and turkey. I remember the first time I cut out grains and dairy it was tough, but the bloating and fatigue I used to feel disappeared. For Type O individuals, high-intensity workouts like running, weightlifting, and martial arts aren't just beneficial; they're essential. We process animal protein efficiently but are prone to thyroid issues, so iodine-rich foods like seaweed are a must. If you're Type O, trust me: this diet can change your life.

Type A: The Cultivator

Now, if you're Type A, your ancestors were the first farmers. This means your body is designed for a vegetarian or plant-based diet. Fresh fruits, vegetables, tofu, and whole grains should be your staples. I've seen friends with Type A blood thrive after switching from heavy meats to plant-based meals. They reported feeling lighter, more energetic, and even sleeping better. The immune system for Type A is more sensitive, so organic foods are essential. Stress management is also crucial; practices like yoga and meditation work wonders. Animal proteins, especially red meat, can cause sluggish digestion, so it's best to avoid them.

Type B: The Nomad

Next up, Type B the most adaptable blood type. Historically, this blood type is linked to nomadic lifestyles, which explains why Type B individuals can tolerate a wider variety of foods. Dairy products, green vegetables, eggs, and certain meats like lamb and venison are all great. However, chicken, corn, wheat, and lentils can disrupt metabolism, leading to fatigue. I had a friend who is Type B, and after cutting out chicken and corn, they noticed a massive energy boost. Moderate exercises like hiking, cycling, and swimming help maintain balance. The flexibility of the Type B diet is ideal for those who don't want a restrictive plan.

Type AB: The Enigma

Type AB is the rarest blood type, combining elements from both A and B. This group is fascinating because it's so new in human history. For AB individuals, a mix of seafood, tofu, dairy, green vegetables, and grains works best. They should avoid red meat, corn, and kidney beans. My cousin, who is AB, found that smaller, more frequent meals worked wonders for their digestion. They also benefit from both calming activities like yoga and moderate exercises like cycling. Because Type AB individuals are more prone to heart disease, maintaining balanced meals and regular exercise is key.

Why Each Type Needs Its Unique Plan

You might wonder, why does this matter? Well, each blood type's unique history affects how we process foods. For instance,

Type O thrives on animal protein, while Type A prefers plant-based meals. """Type B enjoys flexibility but must avoid certain disruptors, and Type AB benefits from a blend of A and B recommendations. Once I understood these differences, it made perfect sense why some diets failed me in the past. Tailoring your diet to your blood type ensures you're working with your body, not against it.

The Role of Exercise in the Blood Type Diet

Exercise isn't one-size-fits-all either. For Type O, high-intensity workouts complement our high-protein diets. Type A individuals should focus on calming exercises that balance their sensitive immune systems. Type B needs moderate activities that reflect their adaptable nature, while Type AB should combine calming and moderate routines. Understanding this connection between diet and exercise can amplify the health benefits of this plan.

Digestion and Metabolism Benefits

Following the right plan can drastically improve digestion and metabolism. I experienced fewer digestive issues after cutting out foods that didn't align with my blood type. My Type A friends had similar results after switching to vegetarian diets. Improved digestion means better nutrient absorption, leading to higher energy levels and better overall health. Tailoring meals this way isn't just about weight loss; it's about holistic wellness.

Stress Management for Each Blood Type

Stress impacts each blood type differently. Type O handles stress through intense physical activity, while Type A needs calming techniques. Type B benefits from mental balance, and Type AB requires a combination of both. Recognizing these patterns helped me adopt stress-relief methods that complemented my dietary changes. Managing stress effectively boosted my energy and helped me stay consistent with the plan.

Common Misconceptions About the Blood Type Diet

Some people dismiss the blood type diet due to a lack of extensive scientific evidence. However, my results speak for themselves. After losing 350 pounds and improving my overall health, I became a believer. The plan's focus on whole, natural foods and personalized exercise regimens makes it a sustainable option. Even if you're skeptical, exploring this diet could reveal insights into your body's needs.

A Personalized Approach to Health

To everyone listening, the blood type diet isn't a quick fix it's a personalized journey. For me, aligning my lifestyle with my Type O blood type was the breakthrough I needed. Whether you're Type A, B, AB, or O, understanding your body's unique requirements can unlock a path to better health, energy, and confidence. Your journey might not mirror mine, but I truly believe this approach can help you discover what works best for you. Give it a try, and your body will thank you.

My Experience with the Type O Blood Type Diet

The Type O blood type diet, also known as the "Hunter's Diet," is considered the oldest and most primal of all blood types. It is believed that this blood type emerged during the hunter-gatherer era, when human ancestors primarily consumed animal protein and lived active lifestyles. Learning about my O positive blood type was a revelation. I realized that my body naturally craved a diet high in lean proteins and low in grains and dairy. This knowledge became the cornerstone of my 350-pound weight-loss journey.

The diet emphasizes the consumption of high-quality, lean proteins such as beef, lamb, turkey, and chicken. These proteins are said to fuel the metabolism of Type O individuals effectively, providing sustained energy and supporting muscle growth. For me, incorporating these foods led to immediate improvements. I no longer felt sluggish after meals, and my digestion improved dramatically. The energy boost I gained from focusing on protein-rich meals motivated me to become more physically active, which further accelerated my weight loss.

Vegetables also play a crucial role in the Type O diet. I prioritized fresh, organic vegetables such as broccoli, spinach, and kale, which provided essential vitamins and minerals. These greens not only supported my digestion but also offered antioxidants that contributed to overall health. On the flip side, I learned to avoid vegetables such as cauliflower and Brussels sprouts, which are thought to interfere with thyroid function in Type O individuals. Making these adjustments improved my metabolism and energy levels, making it easier to stay consistent with my weight loss plan.

Fruits are recommended in moderation for Type O individuals. While I enjoyed fruits like plums, figs, and berries, I avoided oranges and strawberries, which can cause digestive disturbances for those with my blood type. Balancing fruit intake helped me maintain stable blood sugar levels, reducing cravings and preventing energy crashes. This balance was key to sustaining my progress over the long term.

One of the most significant changes I made was eliminating dairy and wheat products. According to the Type O diet, these foods can cause inflammation and hinder weight loss. Before adopting this diet, I often felt bloated and tired after consuming bread, pasta, or dairy products. Once I removed them from my meals, these symptoms disappeared. The reduction in inflammation also relieved joint pain, allowing me to participate in more vigorous physical activities like weightlifting and cardio workouts.

Physical exercise is a vital component of the Type O diet. Our bodies are designed for intense physical activity, mirroring the active lives of ancient hunters. I incorporated high-intensity workouts such as running, strength training, and martial arts. These activities not only burned calories but also improved my cardiovascular health and mental well-being. Exercise became a rewarding routine, enhancing my mood and keeping me motivated throughout my weight loss journey.

Supplements were another essential element of my plan. Type O individuals are prone to thyroid issues, so I included iodine-rich foods such as seaweed and took vitamin K and calcium supplements to support bone health. These additions helped maintain hormonal balance and kept my metabolism running efficiently. With proper supplementation, I experienced fewer plateaus and sustained steady weight loss over the years.

The Type O diet also cautions against certain habits. For example, I learned that caffeine and alcohol can adversely affect cortisol levels, leading to fatigue and weight gain. Reducing my intake of these substances made a noticeable difference in my energy and sleep quality. By focusing on hydration and mindful eating, I felt more in tune with my body's needs, which made sticking to the plan more manageable.

Meal timing played a crucial role as well. I structured my meals to align with my body's natural energy peaks, focusing on larger, protein-rich meals earlier in the day. This approach kept my metabolism active and prevented late-night cravings, which had previously been a significant challenge. Planning and prepping meals in advance became second nature, ensuring I always had nutritious options readily available.

Finally, the mental transformation that accompanied my physical changes was profound. The Type O diet provided a sustainable framework that didn't feel restrictive. As the pounds came off and my energy returned, I regained confidence and a sense of control over my life. My success with the Type O blood type diet is proof that understanding and respecting your body's unique needs can lead to incredible results. For anyone struggling with weight loss, I truly believe that discovering your blood type and aligning your diet accordingly can be life-changing.

Chapter 7

The Importance Of Cardio

Cardiovascular exercises offer numerous physical health benefits that contribute to overall well-being. Here are some key advantages: **Improved Heart Health:** Cardio exercises strengthen the heart muscle, enhancing its efficiency in pumping blood throughout the body. This lowers resting heart rate and improves overall cardiovascular function. **Increased Lung Capacity:** Regular cardio activities improve lung capacity and efficiency, allowing more oxygen to be transported to muscles and organs, thereby enhancing endurance and stamina.

Weight Management: Cardio exercises help burn calories and fat, making them essential for weight loss and weight management when combined with a balanced diet. **Enhanced Circulation:** Cardiovascular workouts promote better blood circulation, reducing the risk of hypertension and improving overall vascular health. **Better Mood:** Cardio releases endorphins, neurotransmitters that improve mood and reduce stress, anxiety, and symptoms of depression. **Improved Sleep:** Regular physical activity, including cardio, promotes deeper, more restful sleep, contributing to overall health and well-being.

Strengthened Immune System: Moderate-intensity cardio exercises can boost the immune system, reducing the risk of chronic diseases and improving overall immune function.

Bone Health: Weight-bearing cardio exercises, such as running, dancing, and hiking, can help maintain bone density and reduce the risk of osteoporosis. **Enhanced Energy Levels:** Regular cardio can increase energy levels by improving the efficiency of the cardiovascular system and enhancing overall physical fitness.

Longevity: Engaging in regular cardio exercises is associated with a longer lifespan and a reduced risk of premature death from cardiovascular disease and other chronic illnesses. Incorporating cardio exercises into your routine not only improves physical health but also enhances mental well-being, contributing to a healthier and more active lifestyle. **Mental Health Benefits:** Exercise is a powerful tool for improving mental health. It can reduce symptoms of depression and anxiety, improve mood, and increase overall mental well-being. Physical activity stimulates the release of endorphins, which are natural mood lifters.

Finding the Right Exercise for You

Choosing an exercise routine that aligns with your personal preferences increases the likelihood of sticking with it. Whether you enjoy running, swimming, dancing, or practicing yoga, finding activities you enjoy makes exercise more sustainable and enjoyable. Your current fitness level and goals should guide your exercise choices. Beginners might start with low-impact activities such as walking or swimming, while those with specific goals, such as building muscle or improving endurance, may opt for weight training or high-intensity interval training (HIIT).

Incorporating a variety of exercises into your routine can prevent boredom and target different muscle groups. Mixing cardio, strength training, and flexibility exercises can keep your workouts balanced and enjoyable. Running and walking are accessible forms of cardio exercise that can be done almost anywhere. They improve cardiovascular health, burn calories, and strengthen the lower body. Adjusting the intensity and duration can help tailor these activities to your fitness level.

Cycling, whether on a stationary bike or outdoors, offers excellent cardiovascular benefits. It is gentle on the joints, making it ideal for those with joint problems, and effectively strengthens the lower body. Swimming is a full-body workout that is easy on the joints. It improves cardiovascular fitness, builds muscle strength, and enhances flexibility. It is an ideal exercise for people of all fitness levels and ages.

The elliptical machine is my favorite fitness machine, offering a low-impact yet effective way to stay active and improve my cardiovascular health. As someone who values joint health, I appreciate that the elliptical provides a smooth, fluid motion that minimizes impact on my knees and hips, making it ideal for my workouts without aggravating any existing joint issues.

One of the aspects I enjoy most about using the elliptical is its ability to engage both my upper and lower body simultaneously. The elliptical handles allow me to work my arms, chest, and back while the pedals engage the muscles in my legs, glutes, and core. This full-body workout not only increases my heart rate for cardiovascular fitness but also helps me burn calories effectively, supporting my overall fitness goals.

The adjustable resistance and incline settings are particularly beneficial, as they allow me to tailor my workouts to different intensities and goals. Whether I'm focusing on endurance, strength, or interval training, I can easily adjust these settings to challenge myself and vary my workout routines. By maintaining proper form, keeping a straight back, engaging my core, and using controlled movements, I ensure that I get the most out of each session while minimizing the risk of injury.

Incorporating Cardio into Your Routine

Cardiovascular exercises are at the forefront of my health routine, offering a multitude of benefits that I find essential for my well-being. These exercises have significantly improved my heart health by strengthening my heart muscle and improving its efficiency in circulating blood. This has helped me manage my blood pressure and maintain healthy cholesterol levels, which are crucial for reducing the risk of heart disease.

Engaging in regular cardio workouts has also been instrumental in managing my weight effectively. By burning calories and creating a calorie deficit, I've been able to achieve and maintain a healthy body weight alongside a balanced diet. Beyond physical health, cardio exercises have a profound impact on my mental well-being. The release of endorphins during workouts boosts my mood, reduces stress, and enhances my overall emotional resilience, which has been invaluable in managing daily life with greater ease.

Moreover, I've noticed a significant increase in my energy levels and stamina since incorporating cardio into my routine. This improvement in cardiovascular efficiency allows me to tackle daily tasks with more vigor and endurance. As someone concerned about long-term health, I appreciate that cardio exercises also contribute to strengthening my bones and supporting bone density, crucial for maintaining skeletal health as I age.

Overall, integrating a variety of cardio activities such as jogging, cycling, and aerobic workouts has not only enhanced my physical fitness but has also provided me with a sense of empowerment and well-being. I aim to maintain at least 150 minutes of moderate-intensity cardio exercise each week, ensuring that I continue to reap the comprehensive benefits of cardio for my long-term health and vitality.

Frequency and Duration

For optimal health benefits, aim for at least 150 minutes of moderate-intensity cardio exercise or 75 minutes of vigorous-intensity exercise per week. This can be broken down into 30-minute sessions, five times a week, or into shorter, more frequent sessions.

Intensity Levels

Adjusting the intensity of your cardio workouts can help you meet your fitness goals. Moderate-intensity activities allow you to talk but not sing during the exercise, while vigorous-intensity activities leave you unable to say more than a few words without pausing for breath. Combining cardio with strength training and flexibility exercises creates a well-rounded fitness routine. This approach ensures that all aspects of fitness are addressed, helping to prevent injuries and improve overall performance.

Chapter 8

Lets Get Stronger

Strength training, also known as resistance training, is essential for overall health and fitness due to its numerous benefits. Firstly, it helps build and maintain muscle mass, which is crucial for everyday activities like lifting objects and maintaining posture. Strong muscles also support joint health, reducing the risk of injuries and improving overall functional ability. Additionally, strength training promotes bone health by increasing bone density and strength, which is particularly important for preventing osteoporosis as we age.

Another significant benefit of strength training is its impact on metabolism and weight management. Muscle tissue burns more calories than fat tissue at rest, so increasing muscle mass through strength training can boost metabolism and aid in fat loss over time. This contributes to a healthier body composition, enhancing physical appearance and boosting self-esteem.

Strength training also improves functional fitness by enhancing balance, flexibility, and coordination. These improvements translate into better performance in daily tasks, sports, and recreational activities, as well as reducing the risk of falls and enhancing overall physical performance. Moreover, regular strength training can help manage chronic conditions such as arthritis, diabetes, and heart disease by improving blood sugar control, cardiovascular health, and overall quality of life.

Lastly, strength training has significant mental health benefits. It stimulates the release of endorphins, promoting feelings of well-being and reducing stress and anxiety. Improved sleep quality and cognitive function are additional mental health benefits associated with regular strength training. Incorporating strength training into a well-rounded fitness routine, alongside cardiovascular exercise and flexibility training, supports overall health and well-being across all stages of life.

Basic Strength Training Exercises

Upper Body Exercises

Upper body exercises are essential for building strength, improving posture, and enhancing functional fitness. Here are some effective upper body exercises you can incorporate into your workout routine:

1. Push-Ups: Targets the chest, shoulders, and triceps. Variations like incline or decline push-ups can adjust the intensity. Pull-

Ups/Chin-Ups: Engages the back, shoulders, and biceps. Use an assisted pull-up machine or resistance bands if needed.

2. Dumbbell Press: Includes exercises like bench press (chest), shoulder press (shoulders), and dumbbell flyes (chest).
3. Bent-Over Rows: Targets the back muscles (lats and rhomboids) using dumbbells or a barbell.
4. Bicep Curls: Focuses on the biceps using dumbbells, barbells, or resistance bands. Variations include hammer curls and concentration curls.
5. Tricep Dips: Works the triceps and shoulders using parallel bars or a sturdy chair.
6. Shoulder Raises: Includes lateral raises (targets the side deltoids), front raises (targets the front deltoids), and rear deltoid raises (targets the rear deltoids).
7. Plank Variations: Engages the core and stabilizes the upper body muscles. Side planks, plank rotations, and forearm planks are effective variations.
8. Overhead Press: Targets the shoulders and triceps using a barbell or dumbbells. Variations include the military press and Arnold press.

9. Chest Press Machine: Offers guided motion for chest workouts, ideal for beginners or those focusing on controlled movements.

Lower Body Exercises

Lower body exercises are essential for building strength, improving balance, and enhancing overall mobility. Here are some effective lower body exercises you can incorporate into your workout routine:

1. Squats: Targets the quadriceps, hamstrings, and glutes. Variations include body-weight squats, goblet squats, and barbell squats.

2. Lunges: Engages the quadriceps, hamstrings, and glutes. Variations include forward lunges, reverse lunges, walking lunges, and lateral lunges.

3. Dead-lifts: Works the hamstrings, glutes, lower back, and core. Variations include conventional dead-lifts, sumo dead-lifts, and Romanian dead-lifts.

4. Leg Press: Targets the quadriceps, hamstrings, and glutes using a leg press machine. Adjust foot position and resistance for different muscle emphasis.

5. Step-Ups: Engage the quadriceps, hamstrings, and glutes. Use a sturdy bench or platform to step up and down, alternating legs.
6. Glute Bridges: Focuses on the glutes and hamstrings. Perform bridges on the floor or use a stability ball for added challenge.
7. Calf Raises: Targets the calves using body weight, dumbbells, or a calf raise machine. Variations include standing calf raises and seated calf raises.
8. Hip Thrusts: Works the glutes, hamstrings, and lower back. Use a bench or stable surface to perform hip thrusts with added resistance.
9. Wall Sits: Engage the quadriceps and glutes. Hold a seated position against a wall for an isometric lower-body workout.
10. Kettlebell Swings: Targets the hips, glutes, and hamstrings. Use a kettlebell to swing from between the legs to chest height in a controlled motion.

When performing lower-body exercises, focus on proper form and technique to prevent injuries and maximize benefits. Start with lighter weights or resistance and gradually increase them as you build strength and confidence. Incorporate a variety of exercises to target different muscle groups for balanced lower-body development. Adjust your workout routine regularly to challenge your muscles and avoid plateaus, and consider consulting a fitness professional for personalized guidance and support.

Core Exercises

Core exercises are crucial for building stability, improving posture, and enhancing overall strength. Here are some effective core exercises you can incorporate into your workout routine:

1. Plank: Engages the entire core, including the abdominals, obliques, and lower back. Hold a plank position on your forearms or hands, maintaining a straight line from head to heels.
2. Crunches: Targets the rectus abdominis (six-pack muscles). Perform standard crunches or variations like bicycle crunches and reverse crunches.
3. Leg Raises: Works the lower abs and hip flexors. Lie on your back and lift your legs toward the ceiling, keeping them straight or bent at the knees.
4. Russian Twists: Engage the obliques and core stability. Sit on the floor, lean back slightly, and rotate your torso from side to side while holding a weight or medicine ball.

5. Mountain Climbers: Combine cardio with core strengthening. Get into a plank position and alternate bringing your knees toward your chest in a running motion.

6. Flutter Kicks: Targets the lower abs and hip flexors. Lie on your back and alternate lifting and lowering your legs in a fluttering motion.

7. Plank Variations: Include side planks (target obliques), forearm planks with hip dips, and planks with shoulder taps for added challenge.

8. Bird Dog: Enhances core stability and balance. Start on your hands and knees, extend one arm forward and the opposite leg backward while keeping your back flat.

9. Bicycle Crunches: Targets the obliques and rectus abdominis. Lie on your back, lift your shoulders off the floor, and bring one knee toward the opposite elbow while extending the other leg.

10. Hanging Leg Raises: Works the lower abs and hip flexors. Hang from a pull-up bar and lift your legs towards your chest or straight out in front of you.

When performing core exercises, focus on maintaining proper form and breathing rhythmically throughout each movement. Start with exercises that match your current fitness level and gradually increase intensity and difficulty as you progress. Incorporate a variety of exercises to target different aspects of core strength and stability for a well-rounded workout routine. Consulting with a fitness professional can provide personalized guidance and help tailor a core workout plan that suits your needs and goals effectively.

Creating a Strength Training Routine

For beginners, aim for at least two strength training sessions per week, focusing on major muscle groups. Each session should include 8-10 different exercises with 1-3 sets of 8-12 repetitions.

Progressive Overload

Progressive overload involves gradually increasing the weight, frequency, or intensity of your exercises to continuously challenge your muscles and promote growth. This can be achieved by adding more weight, increasing the number of repetitions, or reducing rest time between sets.

Recovery and Rest

Rest and recovery are foundational aspects of my fitness journey, essential for achieving my goals while maintaining overall well-being. When I engage in workouts, particularly strength training sessions that challenge my muscles, I recognize the importance of allowing time for muscle repair and growth. Rest days are not just breaks from exercise but crucial opportunities for my body to heal from the stresses of intense physical activity. By prioritizing rest, I ensure that my muscles can recover effectively, allowing me to progress in strength and endurance over time.

Moreover, incorporating rest days into my routine helps me avoid the pitfalls of overtraining. I've learned that pushing myself too hard without adequate recovery can lead to fatigue, decreased motivation, and even injury. By listening to my body and scheduling regular rest days, I prevent burnout and maintain consistency in my workouts. This balance not only improves my physical performance but also enhances my mental resilience and overall enjoyment of fitness.

In terms of performance, I've noticed significant benefits from allowing my muscles to rest and recover. On days when I give my body the time it needs to recuperate, I come back stronger and more energized for my next workout. This cycle of exertion and recovery has been instrumental in improving my strength, endurance, and athletic abilities, ultimately helping me achieve my fitness goals more effectively. Lastly, rest days are a cornerstone of injury prevention in my fitness routine. By taking proactive measures to allow for tissue repair and reduce inflammation, I mitigate the risk of overuse injuries that could sideline my progress. This approach not only supports my physical health but also reinforces my commitment to long-term fitness and well-being.

Chapter 9

Stay Loose On All Ten

Flexibility is a cornerstone of my fitness regimen, playing a vital role in enhancing my overall health and exercise experience. By prioritizing flexibility, I've noticed significant improvements in my range of motion, allowing my joints to move more freely and effectively during workouts. This has not only helped me perform exercises with better form and technique but has also minimized the risk of injuries like muscle strains and ligament sprains that can occur when muscles are tight or overworked.

Moreover, maintaining flexibility contributes to enhanced performance across various types of physical activities. Whether I'm lifting weights, running, or engaging in sports, flexible muscles and tendons enable me to generate more power and strength, leading to better athletic performance and endurance. This aspect of flexibility has been instrumental in pushing my fitness boundaries and achieving new personal goals.

Beyond physical benefits, flexibility exercises have a profound impact on my posture and alignment. Regular stretching helps lengthen tight muscles that can pull the body out of alignment, improving my overall posture and reducing the likelihood of chronic pain associated with poor posture habits. This focus on alignment not only supports my physical health but also enhances my comfort and confidence during everyday movements and activities.

Additionally, incorporating flexibility into my routine promotes relaxation and aids in quicker muscle recovery post-workout. Stretching sessions serve as moments of mindfulness and stress relief, contributing to my overall mental well-being. By integrating stretching and flexibility exercises into my fitness routine consistently, I'm able to maintain joint health, reduce muscle tension, and support my long-term fitness journey effectively.

Flexibility-promoting workouts encompass a variety of exercises and activities designed to enhance range of motion, reduce muscle stiffness, and improve overall mobility. These workouts emphasize stretching and lengthening muscles and tendons, crucial for maintaining flexibility and preventing injuries. Static stretching is a fundamental technique in which muscles are stretched to a point of mild discomfort and held for a specified duration, typically 15-30 seconds per stretch. This method targets specific muscle groups like hamstrings, quadriceps, and calves, effectively improving flexibility over time.

Dynamic stretching involves controlled movements that take joints and muscles through a full range of motion. Unlike static stretching, dynamic stretches are active and help improve flexibility while also warming up the body for physical activity. Examples include leg swings, arm circles, and walking lunges with a twist, which prepare muscles and joints for exercise while promoting flexibility.

Yoga stands out as a comprehensive practice that combines physical postures (asanas), breathing techniques, and meditation. It promotes flexibility, strength, and balance through a series of poses that stretch and lengthen muscles. Poses like downward dog, warrior poses, and seated forward folds not only increase flexibility but also enhance overall body awareness and relaxation.

Pilates focuses on core strength, stability, and flexibility through controlled movements that emphasize proper alignment and muscle engagement. It targets muscles in the abdomen, back, hips, and shoulders, improving flexibility in these areas while promoting overall body conditioning. Tai Chi, an ancient Chinese martial art, incorporates slow, flowing movements and deep breathing exercises that enhance flexibility, balance, and relaxation. Its gentle, meditative approach makes it suitable for individuals of all fitness levels.

Best Ways for Beginners to Get More Flexible

Flexibility is a crucial component of overall fitness, enhancing mobility, posture, and balance while reducing the risk of injury. Whether you're young or old, male or female, improving flexibility can lead to better performance in daily activities and workouts. Here's an expanded and highly detailed breakdown of how beginners can enhance flexibility, focusing on each major body group with tailored advice for different ages and genders.

The neck and shoulders often hold tension from daily activities like sitting at a desk or using electronic devices. For all age groups, slow neck tilts and rotations, along with shoulder blade squeezes, are fundamental starting points. The Thread the Needle pose from yoga relieves shoulder tension, and a wall shoulder stretch helps open up tight shoulders.

For older adults, gentle shoulder shrugs while seated can support safe mobility, while younger individuals can benefit from yoga sun salutations. Males may gain from resistance band shoulder stretches, while females might try shoulder circles with light dumbbells for toned, flexible shoulders.

Tightness in the upper back and chest can lead to poor posture and breathing restrictions.

Beginners can lie back on a stability ball with arms extended to stretch the chest or use a wall chest stretch by leaning forward in a doorway. For those seeking more challenge, the Bow Pose from yoga or a foam roller chest opener offers deeper stretches. Older adults can try seated chest openers with support, and younger individuals might include bridge poses. Males should perform pec stretches after upper-body workouts, while females can include gentle yoga sequences focusing on the chest and upper back.

Flexibility in the arms and wrists supports everyday activities like lifting and typing. Beginners can extend an arm with the palm up and gently pull back on the fingers to stretch the wrists, complemented by overhead triceps stretches. Yoga's plank-to-downward-dog sequence helps stretch the arms while building strength. Finger extensions help maintain dexterity, especially for older adults. Males should integrate biceps stretches using resistance bands, while females benefit from wrist flexion and extension routines, especially if they practice yoga regularly.

A flexible core and lower back enhance stability and prevent injury. Spinal twists, performed by placing the opposite hand on the knee while seated, increase flexibility. Yoga poses like Cobra and Sphinx enhance spinal extension. For added variety, the bird-dog exercise strengthens and stretches the core, while a foam roller back stretch loosens tight muscles. Older adults can start with seated spinal rotations, while younger individuals may enjoy side planks for oblique flexibility. Males can focus on weighted side bends, and females might combine hip bridges with lower back stretches for a balanced routine.

Flexible hips and glutes are vital for mobility and lower-body strength. The lying figure-four stretch, where one ankle crosses over the opposite knee, is a gentle starting point. Lunging forward with one leg while the other knee rests on the ground stretches the hip flexor. More advanced beginners can explore Frog Pose or Happy Baby Pose for deeper hip openings. Standing hip swings work well for older adults, while younger individuals can incorporate lunges with spinal rotation. Males might target a tighter hip flexor with deep lunges, and females can benefit from the butterfly pose for pelvic flexibility.

Flexible legs contribute to balance and functional movement. Beginners can try seated forward folds by reaching for their toes or standing quad stretches by pulling the foot toward the glutes. Downward Dog stretches the calves, hamstrings, and spine, while a wall calf stretch targets the lower legs. Chair-assisted hamstring stretches provide safe options for older adults. Dynamic hamstring stretches before workouts benefit younger individuals. Males should consider calf raises after stretching for strength, and females might add the dancer's pose for balance and flexibility.

Flexible ankles and feet support balance and mobility, crucial for all movement. Beginners can perform toe spreads while seated or heel walks to strengthen and stretch the ankles. Foot flexes using resistance bands improve arch flexibility and the Achilles tendon stretch, done by leaning into a wall with one leg extended and supporting the lower leg. Gentle ankle pumps work well for older adults, while younger individuals might enjoy jump rope for dynamic flexibility. Males benefit from Achilles stretches, especially if they engage in running, while females can focus on yoga poses that support the foot arch.

Advanced flexibility practices for beginners include dynamic stretching with leg swings and arm circles before workouts. Partner stretching, when done with proper guidance, can enhance flexibility. The contract-and-relax technique in PNF stretching allows for deeper stretches. Yoga and Pilates classes offer structured full-body flexibility, while Tai Chi's gentle movements are ideal for older adults looking to improve flexibility and balance.

When improving flexibility, warming up with light cardio is essential to prevent injury. Deep breathing helps muscles relax during stretching sessions. Consistency is key; daily 10-15 minute sessions yield steady progress. Moving gently and avoiding forced stretches allows flexibility to develop gradually. Staying hydrated and properly nourished supports muscle elasticity.

Regardless of age or gender, improving flexibility enhances quality of life. With consistent effort and a tailored approach, anyone can achieve greater mobility, reduced pain, and improved physical performance, leading to a healthier, more active lifestyle.

Foam rolling involves using a foam roller to apply pressure to tight or sore muscles. This technique helps release knots and adhesions in muscle tissue, reducing muscle tension and improving flexibility. Stretching classes and dance styles like ballet and contemporary dance also contribute to flexibility through dynamic movements and stretches that target various muscle groups.

Incorporating these flexibility-promoting workouts into a regular fitness routine can yield significant benefits, including increased range of motion, reduced risk of injuries, and improved overall mobility. Whether through dedicated stretching sessions, yoga practice, or dynamic warm-ups before exercise, prioritizing flexibility helps maintain muscle health and supports long-term physical well-being. Regular practice and gradual progression in stretching techniques ensure safe and effective improvement in flexibility over time, enhancing both athletic performance and everyday movement capabilities.

Chapter 10

Make
a
Plan

Assessing Your Fitness Level

Before starting a workout plan, assess your current fitness level. This can include measuring your weight, body composition, cardiovascular endurance, muscular strength, and flexibility. Fitness assessments can be performed at a gym, with a personal trainer, at home, or using online resources.

How to Perform a Fitness Assessment at Home

A home fitness assessment is a great way to evaluate your current physical condition, set realistic goals, and track progress over time. By conducting simple tests, you can measure various aspects of fitness, including cardiovascular endurance, muscular strength, flexibility, and body composition. Here's a step-by-step guide to conducting a detailed fitness assessment at home.

Before starting, choose a quiet, comfortable space with enough room for movement. Wear athletic clothing and shoes, have a stopwatch or a smartphone timer, and keep a notebook or a fitness tracking app to record your results. Warm up for five to ten minutes with light cardio and dynamic stretching to prepare your muscles and joints for testing.

Measuring Body Composition

Body composition refers to the proportion of fat, muscle, bone, and water in your body. You can measure it in several ways: Body Weight: Use a digital scale to record your weight at the same time of day, preferably in the morning before eating or drinking. **Body Mass Index (BMI):** Calculate your BMI by dividing your weight by your height squared. While BMI does not differentiate between fat and muscle, it provides a general indication of whether your weight is in a healthy range.

Waist-to-Hip Ratio: Measure your waist circumference at the narrowest point and your hip circumference at the widest part. Divide your waist measurement by your hip measurement to assess fat distribution and potential health risks. Skin-Fold **Measurements:** If available, use calipers to measure skin-fold thickness at key areas (abdomen, triceps, thigh) to estimate body fat percentage.

Ready Set Test

Cardiovascular Endurance Test - Cardiovascular endurance measures how well your heart and lungs supply oxygen to your body during prolonged exercise. Try the following tests:

3-Minute Step Test: Use a 12-inch step and step up and down at a consistent pace for three minutes. After finishing, check your pulse for one full minute and compare it to standard recovery heart-rate charts.

1-Mile Walk Test: Walk one mile as quickly as possible, then measure your heart rate immediately afterward. This test indicates aerobic fitness and stamina. Running Test: If you prefer, run for 12 minutes (Cooper Test) and measure the distance covered. The further you run, the higher your cardiovascular fitness.

Muscular Strength and Endurance Test: These tests evaluate how much force your muscles can exert and their ability to sustain repeated contractions.

Push-Up Test: Perform as many push-ups as possible in one minute. Modify by doing knee push-ups if needed. This test assesses upper body strength and endurance. Plank Hold: Hold a plank position for as long as possible while maintaining proper form. This measures core strength and endurance.

- **Squat Test:** Perform as many body-weight squats as possible in one minute to assess lower-body strength.

- **Wall Sit Test:** Sit against a wall with your knees at 90 degrees and hold the position for as long as possible.
- **Flexibility Assessment -** Flexibility tests measure the range of motion in your muscles and joints.
- **Sit-and-Reach Test:** Sit on the floor with your legs extended and reach forward toward your toes. Measure how far you can stretch.
- **Shoulder Flexibility Test:** Try to touch your hands together behind your back by reaching one hand over your shoulder and the other up from your lower back. This assesses shoulder mobility.
- **Hip Flexor Stretch Test:** Lie on a flat surface and pull one knee toward your chest while keeping the other leg extended. If the extended leg lifts, it may indicate tight hip flexors.
- **Balance and Coordination Test -** Balance and coordination are essential for functional movement and injury prevention.
- **Single-Leg Stand Test:** Stand on one foot with your eyes open for as long as possible. Repeat with your eyes closed for an advanced challenge.

- **Heel-to-Toe Walk:** Walk in a straight line, placing the heel of one foot directly in front of the toes of the other. This evaluates coordination and stability.

Once you've completed your home fitness assessment, record all results in a notebook or digital app. Compare your results to standard fitness norms for your age and gender, if available. Repeat the assessment every four to six weeks to track improvements and adjust your workout plan accordingly. If any test feels uncomfortable or causes pain, stop immediately. Use the results to create a tailored fitness plan that suits your strengths and areas for improvement. A home fitness assessment is a valuable tool for understanding your fitness level and setting realistic goals. By regularly evaluating your progress, you can stay motivated and make informed adjustments to your exercise routine, ensuring steady improvement over time.

Based on your fitness assessment, set specific, measurable, achievable, relevant, and time-bound (SMART) goals. Whether your aim is to lose weight, gain muscle, improve endurance, or enhance overall fitness, having clear goals will guide your workout plan. A balanced workout routine includes cardio, strength training, and flexibility exercises. Aim for at least 150 minutes of moderate-intensity cardio per week, two to three strength training sessions, and regular stretching or yoga sessions.

Create a weekly workout schedule that fits your lifestyle. For example, you might do cardio on Monday, Wednesday, and Friday, strength training on Tuesday and Thursday, and yoga or stretching on Saturday. Ensure you have at least one rest day per week. Pay attention to your body's signals and adjust your workout plan as needed. If you experience pain, fatigue, or signs of overtraining, consider modifying your exercises, reducing intensity, or taking extra rest days. Regularly track your progress to stay motivated and make necessary adjustments to your plan. Use a fitness journal, app, or wearable device to record your workouts, monitor your performance, and celebrate your achievements.

Chapter 11

So You Plateaued?

What is a plateau?

A plateau occurs when your progress stalls despite consistent efforts. In weight loss, this means you stop losing weight even though you're following your diet and exercise plan. Plateaus are common and can be frustrating, but they are a natural part of the weight loss journey. Plateaus can be caused by various factors, including metabolic adaptation, changes in body composition, overtraining, or a lack of variety in your routine. Understanding the underlying causes can help you break through them.

Adjusting Caloric Intake

Reassess your caloric needs and adjust your intake if necessary. As you lose weight, your body requires fewer calories. Consider reducing your caloric intake slightly or incorporating a calorie cycling approach, where you vary your daily intake to keep your metabolism active. Introduce new exercises, increase intensity, or change your workout routine to challenge your body in different ways. Adding intervals, trying new cardio activities, or incorporating different strength training techniques can help overcome plateaus. Stalls and variations in weight can happen, and there's nothing to be particularly alarmed about unless you notice rapid losses and gains. You should consult your healthcare professional immediately if this happens.

Weight Variations

It's normal for weight to fluctuate daily and weekly due to factors such as fluid balance, food intake, and hormonal changes. Understanding that these fluctuations are part of the body's natural processes can help you avoid frustration. High sodium intake can cause temporary water retention, leading to weight fluctuations. Similarly, carbohydrates bind to water, so changes in carbohydrate intake can affect water weight. Monitoring sodium and carbohydrate consumption can help manage these fluctuations. Instead of fixating on daily weight changes, focus on long-term trends. Use weekly or monthly averages to track your progress and understand that small fluctuations are normal and do not indicate failure.

Rewards and Incentives

One of the biggest lessons I've learned on my weight loss journey is that rewarding progress in a healthy way is just as important as staying disciplined. Many people, myself included, have fallen into the habit of using food as a reward, which can create an unhealthy cycle of emotional eating and sabotage long-term success. Instead of indulging in junk food every time I reach a milestone, I've found that choosing non-food rewards that support my health and fitness goals keeps me motivated while reinforcing positive habits. For instance, investing in new workout gear, such as high-quality running shoes, stylish gym clothes, or resistance bands, gives me something to look forward to while also encouraging me to stay active.

A self-care session, such as a massage, a manicure & pedicure, or even a relaxing bath with Epsom salts, helps me unwind and reward myself without derailing progress. I also love treating myself to fitness gadgets like a smart water bottle, a high-speed blender for healthy smoothies, or an air fryer to make meal prep easier and more enjoyable. Beyond material rewards, I've discovered that experiences such as trying a new fitness class, planning a weekend hike, or going for a beach run are incredibly fulfilling and reinforce the joy of movement and self-improvement.

When it comes to cheat days, I've learned the hard way that indulging for an entire day can quickly erase a week's worth of progress, leading to bloating, sluggishness, and blood sugar spikes that make it harder to get back on track. Instead, I follow a more balanced approach by allowing myself one planned cheat meal per week rather than an all-day binge. This strategy lets me satisfy cravings without feeling guilty or sabotaging my goals.

To keep my cheat meals under control, I always plan ahead, deciding in advance what I'll indulge in so that I don't let emotions or impulsivity take over. I also practice portion control, enjoying my favorite foods in moderation rather than overindulging to the point of discomfort. If I'm having something high in carbs or fat, like pizza or pasta, I make sure to balance it with protein and fiber, such as by adding a grilled chicken salad on the side, to slow digestion and prevent a blood sugar crash.

Another key habit I've developed is staying hydrated before and after my cheat meal to reduce bloating and flush out excess sodium. I also try to incorporate my cheat meal into my overall calorie intake, so it doesn't completely throw me off track. Instead of a 3,000-calorie binge, I enjoy my indulgence while still being mindful of my limits. Most importantly, I've learned that getting back on track immediately after a cheat meal is crucial. I no longer let one indulgence turn into a downward spiral. I enjoy my treats guilt-free and return to my usual healthy eating habits right afterward.

By shifting my mindset to rewarding progress in a way that aligns with my fitness goals, I've been able to stay consistent and motivated without feeling deprived. Healthy rewards, combined with controlled cheat meals, allow me to enjoy the journey while still making sustainable progress. This balance has helped me develop a healthier relationship with food, making weight loss feel like a lifestyle rather than a temporary diet.

Incorporating healthy rewards and strategic cheat meals can absolutely help break through weight loss plateaus by boosting metabolism, reducing stress, and increasing motivation. When weight loss stalls, it's often due to the body adapting to a routine, slowing metabolism, or holding onto water weight due to prolonged calorie restriction. Strategic rewards and controlled indulgences can help reset the body, regulate hormones, and re-ignite progress without derailing results.

One major reason plateaus occur is that prolonged calorie restriction causes metabolic adaptation, meaning the body becomes more efficient at using fewer calories, making it harder to lose weight. A well-planned cheat meal or calorie refeed can actually help reset metabolism by signaling to the body that it's not in a state of starvation. When I strategically incorporate a cheat meal that includes healthy carbs and protein, such as sushi, whole-grain pasta, or a burger with a lettuce wrap, it can temporarily boost leptin levels, the hormone responsible for regulating hunger and fat metabolism. This brief increase in calories can help kick-start fat burning again by preventing the body from going into energy conservation mode.

Additionally, rewarding myself with fitness-related incentives keeps me motivated and engaged rather than feeling stuck in a frustrating cycle. When I hit a plateau, rather than getting discouraged, I shift my focus to non-scale victories like strength gains, endurance improvements, and changes.

Another way that cheat meals and healthy rewards can help break a plateau is by reducing mental burnout. Sticking to a strict diet for too long can cause diet fatigue, making it harder to stay disciplined. When I give myself permission to enjoy a planned treat guilt-free, it prevents binge-eating episodes, which often happen when restriction is too severe. However, I always plan my cheat meals intentionally. I don't use them as an excuse to overeat, but rather as a way to reset my mindset, satisfy cravings, and prevent long-term cravings from turning into uncontrolled binges.

Incorporating healthy rewards and planned cheat meals strategically is a powerful tool for breaking plateaus. It keeps metabolism active, prevents diet fatigue, reduces stress-related weight retention, and helps me stay motivated even when progress slows. Instead of feeling discouraged, I see plateaus as an opportunity to reevaluate, refresh, and re-ignite my weight loss journey in a way that is sustainable and enjoyable.

Chapter 12

Celebrate Every Milestone

The Power of Celebrating Every Milestone on a Weight Loss Journey

One of the most important lessons I've learned on my weight loss journey is the importance of **celebrating every milestone**, no matter how small. Too often, people focus only on the final goal, whether it's a certain number on the scale, a specific clothing size, or an ideal body shape. But the truth is that weight loss and health transformations are long-term journeys, and recognizing progress along the way is what keeps me motivated, inspired, and committed. Every step forward, no matter how small, is proof that I am improving, growing, and getting closer to my best self.

Acknowledging milestones helps maintain motivation and prevents burnout. When I started my journey, I used to feel discouraged when I didn't see drastic changes right away. But as I began **celebrating smaller victories**, like drinking more water daily, resisting emotional eating, lifting heavier weights, or simply being more consistent with my workouts, I realized that progress isn't just about the scale. Seeing these changes gave me a sense of accomplishment and helped me stay excited about the process rather than feeling like I was endlessly chasing a distant goal.

Another key reason to celebrate every milestone is that it **reinforces positive behaviors**. Weight loss isn't just about losing pounds; it's about building habits that support a healthier lifestyle. Every time I acknowledge progress, it strengthens my motivation to keep going. For example, when I noticed that I could jog for an extra five minutes without stopping, it made me want to push even further. When I saw my clothes fitting better, I felt more confident and excited to keep going. These moments serve as **fuel for perseverance**, keeping me committed even when progress slows.

Celebrating milestones also helps shift focus away from just numbers on the scale. Non-scale victories, such as increased energy levels, better sleep, clearer skin, improved endurance, and a more positive mindset, are just as important as weight loss itself. When I focus on these victories, I recognize that my efforts are paying off in ways beyond appearance. This makes my journey feel more fulfilling, holistic, and meaningful.

To make the most of these celebrations, I've learned to **reward myself in ways that align with my health goals**. Instead of turning to food as a reward, I celebrate progress with things that enhance my journey, such as **buying new activewear, treating myself, investing in a fitness gadget, signing up for a fun activity, or setting a new personal challenge**. These rewards reinforce my progress without setting me back.

Most importantly, **celebrating every milestone keeps me focused on the bigger picture**. Weight loss isn't a race; it's a lifestyle change. Recognizing my achievements along the way reminds me that every step forward matters, and the effort I put in each day is building a stronger, healthier version of myself. By appreciating each moment of progress, big or small, I stay inspired, confident, and committed to becoming the best version of myself.

Celebrating milestones in unique and meaningful ways can keep motivation high while reinforcing positive habits. One powerful way to acknowledge progress is by creating a visual progress board or collage filled with photos, quotes, and reminders of how far I've come. Seeing my transformation visually can be incredibly inspiring and serve as a daily reminder of my dedication. Another fun way to celebrate is by planning a themed photo shoot, where I can dress up in an outfit that makes me feel confident or even showcase my fitness journey. These personal photos serve as a great way to document my progress and boost my self-esteem.

For a more adventurous celebration, I love stepping out of my comfort zone by trying a new challenge or experience, such as rock climbing, zip-lining, or paddle-boarding. These activities not only make the milestone memorable but also reinforce the idea that my body is capable of new and exciting things. A deeply personal way to celebrate is by getting a small symbolic tattoo or custom jewelry engraved with a meaningful mantra, date, or word that represents my journey. It serves as a lasting reminder of how much I've grown, both mentally and physically. Another creative idea is to throw a personal "fitness graduation" celebration, where I invite close friends and family to share in my success. It doesn't have to be extravagant; just a small gathering to recognize my hard work and dedication.

Transforming my personal space can also serve as a great reward. Upgrading my bedroom or living area with new decor, fresh bedding, or a wellness corner filled with yoga mats, candles, and affirmations can symbolize my new, healthier lifestyle. If I want a more relaxing celebration, I might book a wellness session, such as acupuncture, or a deep-tissue massage to relieve stress and rejuvenate my body. Another meaningful way to document my progress is by creating a "before and after" scrapbook with journal entries, photos, and small souvenirs from my journey. Reading about my past struggles and triumphs reminds me of how strong and resilient I've become.

A deeply reflective way to celebrate is by writing a letter to my future self, describing my current emotions, struggles, and victories. I can open it at my next milestone to see how much I've evolved. If I want to treat myself to something luxurious, booking a hot air balloon ride, a weekend retreat, or a VIP concert ticket provides an unforgettable experience that rewards my hard work. Another confidence-boosting celebration is getting a new haircut or makeover, symbolizing a fresh start and the transformation I've undergone.

Perhaps the most fulfilling way to celebrate is by giving back to others who are starting their own fitness journey. You can donate workout gear to someone in need, support a fitness-related charity, or mentor a friend who's struggling with their goals. Helping others reminds me of where I started and gives my journey a greater purpose. By celebrating milestones in creative, non-food ways, I not only keep myself motivated but also reinforce self-love, gratitude, and long-term success. Every milestone, no matter how small, deserves to be recognized because each step forward is a victory worth celebrating.

A Journey of Healing and Transformation

As this book comes to a close, I want to take a moment to express my deepest gratitude to you, the reader. Thank you for taking the time to embark on this journey of self-discovery, growth, and transformation. Whether you came here seeking guidance, motivation, or simply a new perspective, I hope that the words within these pages have ignited something powerful within you.

Your journey, both mental and physical, is uniquely yours, and no matter where you are in the process, I want you to know that healing is possible. True transformation goes beyond weight loss, fitness routines, or meal plans; it is about learning to love yourself, honoring your progress, and embracing every challenge as an opportunity to grow. It is about breaking free from the cycles that have held you back, reclaiming your strength, and stepping fully into the life you deserve.

I encourage you to take everything you have learned here and apply it with patience, self-compassion, and consistency. The road ahead may not always be easy, but every step forward, no matter how small, is a victory. Celebrate your progress, embrace the lessons in the setbacks, and, most importantly, never give up on yourself.

I hope that in these pages, you have found not just information but inspiration, encouragement, and a renewed sense of hope. May you continue to move forward with confidence, knowing that you are worthy of healing, happiness, and a life of fulfillment. Keep striving, keep believing, and, most of all, keep becoming the best version of yourself.

With gratitude and encouragement,

Quanjay J. Jones

Outro

As you embark on your journey toward better health and well-being, the workbook and meal plan are designed to support you every step of the way. Whether you're looking for guidance on understanding your body's needs or seeking practical, actionable steps to transform your diet, these resources are here to help. The workbook delves into the principles of healthy eating, goal-setting, and tracking progress, while the meal plan provides you with a structured, balanced approach to fueling your body. Both can be purchased separately, allowing you to choose the resource that best fits your current needs. Together or individually, they are tools to empower you on your path to a healthier, more vibrant life.

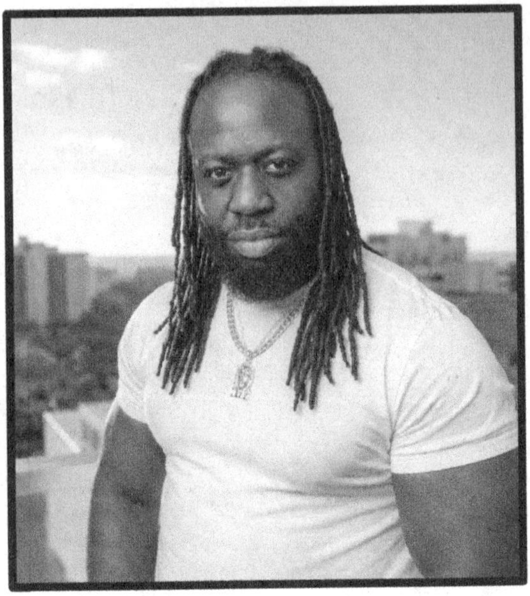

About the Author

Quanjay Joculb Jones is a multifaceted individual with a passion for helping others achieve their full potential. Born and raised in Columbia, South Carolina, Quanjay's life has been shaped by personal experiences that have inspired his pursuit of health, wellness, and mental growth. Having overcome adversity, including the struggles of growing up in poverty and enduring trauma, Quanjay has used these challenges as fuel to drive his commitment to personal development and self-empowerment.

In addition to his work as a Christian Hip Hop artist under the stage name

Quanjay Lyon, Quanjay is a seasoned ministry leader, dedicating over 15 years to empowering individuals through powerful teachings and revelations. His life experiences have given him a deep understanding of the importance of both mental and physical well-being, and he channels this wisdom into his work, including his music, books, and lifestyle coaching.

Quanjay has written numerous literary works, including his first album *Molested Minds* and his book *They Molested My Mind - The Power Of A Choice*, which explore his journey of survival, healing, and faith. His diverse background in music, ministry, and personal growth serves as the foundation for his unique approach to helping others improve their lives, both physically and spiritually.

Through his experiences, Quanjay has developed a strong belief that the path to true health involves more than just physical fitness. It's about healing the mind, nurturing the soul, and building a resilient mindset. His work, including this book, is a reflection of his dedication to guiding others toward holistic wellness and encouraging them to face their challenges with strength, courage, and unwavering faith.

Whether through his music, books, or personal coaching, Quanjay continues to inspire and motivate individuals to overcome their obstacles, pursue their passions, and transform their lives into something they are proud of.

Made in the USA
Coppell, TX
05 November 2026

11315637R20099